CHAPTER 1

The Nurse as Communicator

Communication—perhaps the most used and abused word in nursing. Few, if any, would deny nurses need effective communication skills. However, what communication skills do nurses need? How do nurses acquire these skills? Perhaps an even more important question is, if nurses possess communication skills, will they be better nurses?

A simple answer to all these questions is: it depends. Each of you as a nurse functions in situations which place unique communicative demands upon you. The specific skills needed to meet these demands are as varied as the situations you encounter. While needed specific skills may vary, there are some ways of thinking about communication that we believe all of you can enact to become more competent communicators.

Before you can "live" effective nursing communication, we must first briefly explore a few aspects of the career each of you has chosen—a career within the nursing community.

PROFESSIONAL IMAGE OF NURSING

Many have viewed nursing as a semi- or quasi-profession. Nurses were viewed as subservient to physicians and other "professionals," expected to simply follow orders and provide necessary technical skills to aid the health care process. During the past two decades, this view of nursing has been undergoing change. Because of societal barriers and obstacles created by nurses themselves, progress in changing the nurse's image, however, has been slow.

The view of nursing as a profession has been hindered by a view of nursing as requiring a lower educational level than other professions, mass media's portrayal of nurses as nonprofessional, reluctant acceptance of the nurse's intellectual knowledge and abilities by allied professionals, the varying educational backgrounds of nurses, and the nurse's own self-perceptions.

The nursing community recognizes these image problems and has been working to solve them. For example, through organized efforts and protests by nurses, the image of nurses in the media has become more positive, although even as of this writing, some "media nurses" are depicted as less than professional. The April 1982 issue of *The American Nurse* reports that *Playboy* magazine cancelled a proposed photo session featuring registered nurses because of the initiative by a St. Louis hospital RN and the Missouri Nurses Association. Although *Playboy*'s editors stated their layout was scrapped because the photographs were of poor quality and scheduling problems, they acknowledged being deluged with letters and phone calls protesting the potential "negative image of the nursing profession" the photo section could project.

Other image "solutions" focus on increasing and standardizing formal educational requirements for nurses. For example, the American Nurse's Association (ANA) has advocated the baccalaureate as a professional requirement since 1965 and has become extremely active in support of this position since its convention in 1978.* More and more nursing organizations have added their support to the ANA position. In 1982, *The American Nurse* reported that the board of directors of the National League for Nursing (NLN) adopted a position statement calling for the B.S.N. degree as the academic preparation for professional nursing practice, and the American Association of Critical Care Nurses adopted a similar position.

The NLN statement distinguished vocational, technical, and professional nurses and stated that, in their opinion, preparation for vocational nursing requires a certificate or diploma in vocational/practical nursing, preparation for technical nursing practice requires an associate degree or a diploma in nursing, and preparation for professional nursing requires a baccalaureate degree with a major in nursing.

While enactment of the ANA Resolution is uncertain at this time, it is our belief that even if legislated, the ANA Resolution will not by itself remove the barriers to a more positive nursing image. It is doubtful, in

---

*The ANA "1985 Resolution" calls for a baccalaureate (B.S.N.) degree as an entry level requirement for licensure of "professional nurses" after 1985.

The Scott, Foresman PROCOM Series

Series Editors

Roderick P. Hart
University of Texas at Austin

Ronald L. Applbaum
Pan American University

Titles in the PROCOM Series

BETTER WRITING FOR PROFESSIONALS
A Concise Guide
Carol Gelderman

BETWEEN YOU AND ME
The Professional's Guide to Interpersonal Communication
Robert Hopper
In consultation with Lillian Davis

COMMUNICATION STRATEGIES FOR TRIAL ATTORNEYS
K. Phillip Taylor
Raymond W. Buchanan
David U. Strawn

THE CORPORATE MANAGER'S GUIDE TO BETTER COMMUNICATION
W. Charles Redding
In consultation with Michael Z. Sincoff

GETTING THE JOB DONE
A Guide to Better Communication for Office Staff
Bonnie M. Johnson
In consultation with Geri Sherman

THE MILITARY OFFICER'S GUIDE TO BETTER COMMUNICATION
L. Brooks Hill
In consultation with Major Michael Gallagher

THE NURSE'S GUIDE TO BETTER COMMUNICATION
Robert E. Carlson
In consultation with Margaret Kidwell Udin and Mary Carlson

THE PHYSICIAN'S GUIDE TO BETTER COMMUNICATION
Barbara F. Sharf
In consultation with Dr. Joseph A. Flaherty

THE POLICE OFFICER'S GUIDE TO BETTER COMMUNICATION
T. Richard Cheatham
Keith V. Erickson
In consultation with Frank Dyson

PROFESSIONALLY SPEAKING
A Concise Guide
Robert J. Doolittle
In consultation with Thomas Towers

For further information, write to

Professional Publishing Group
Scott, Foresman and Company
1900 East Lake Avenue
Glenview, IL 60025

The Nurse's Guide to Better Communication

PROCOM

SERIES EDITORS

Roderick P. Hart
University of Texas at Austin

Ronald L. Applbaum
Pan American University

The Nurse's Guide to Better Communication

Robert E. Carlson, Ph.D.
University of Nebraska at Omaha

in consultation with
Margaret Kidwell Udin, R.N.
Meyer Children's Institute, Omaha

Mary Louise Carlson, R.N.
Creighton University School of Nursing, Omaha

Scott, Foresman and Company   Glenview, Illinois
Dallas, Texas   Oakland, New Jersey   Palo Alto, California
Tucker, Georgia   London

ACKNOWLEDGMENTS

(Figure 8—The Social Penetration Process) From Irwin Altman and Dalmas A. Taylor, *Social Penetration: The Development of Interpersonal Relationships*, p. 17, 1973, Holt, Rinehart & Winston, Inc. Copyright by Professor Irwin Altman.   Adapted from *Nonverbal Communication in Human Interaction*, second edition, by Mark L. Knapp. Copyright © 1978 by Holt, Rinehart & Winston. Reprinted by permission of Holt, Rinehart & Winston, CBS College Publishing. From *Communication Within the Organization* by W. Charles Redding. Copyright © 1972 by Purdue Research Foundation, West Lafayette, Indiana 47907. Reprinted with permission.   From *Principles and Types of Speech*, 6th ed., by Alan H. Monroe and Douglas Ehninger. Copyright © 1967 by Scott, Foresman and Company.

Library of Congress Cataloging in Publication Data

Carlson, Robert E.
  The nurse's guide to better communication.

  Includes bibliographies and index.
  1. Communication in nursing.   2. Interpersonal
communication.   I. Title. [DNLM: 1. Communication—
Nursing texts. 2. Nurse—Patient relations. 3. Inter-
professional relations. WY 87 C2845n]
RT23.C37   1984   610.73'06'99   83-11704
ISBN 0-673-15552-8

Copyright © 1984 Scott, Foresman and Company.
All Rights Reserved.
Printed in the United States of America.

1 2 3 4 5 6 - MAL - 88 87 86 85 84 83

CONTENTS

FOREWORD ix

PREFACE xi

CHAPTER 1
The Nurse as Communicator 1

Professional Image of Nursing 1
Nurses as Professional 3
A Definition of Communication for Nurses 4
The Role of Nursing and Communication 7
Nursing Communicative Competence 12
Communicative Attitude Sets 13
Nursing Professionalism and Rhetorical Sensitivity 21
Summary 22

CHAPTER 2
The Nurse as Interviewer 26

A Definition of an Interview 26
Your Involvement in Nursing Interviews 29
Interviewing Strategies Available to Nurses 32
Implementation of Nursing Interview Strategies 34
Nonverbal Communication 42
Summary 50

CHAPTER 3
Communicating with Patients 53

Communicative Needs of Patients/Clients 53
Your Responsibilities in Nurse/Patient Interviews 58
Conduct and Analysis of Actual Nurse/Patient Interviews 59
Nurse/Patient Interviewing Exercises 63
Summary 74

CHAPTER 4
Communicating with Health Care Professionals 76

Nonpatient Nursing Interviews 76
Nursing Small Group Communication 86
Summary 95

CHAPTER 5
Communicating in Health Care Organizations and Public Speaking 98

Nursing and Organizational Communication 98
The Nurse as Public Communicator 106
Summary 120

INDEX 123

FOREWORD

This volume is part of a series entitled *ProCom* (Professional Communication), which has been created to bring the very latest thinking about human communication to the attention of working professionals. Busy professionals rarely have time for theoretical writings on communication oriented toward general readers, and the books in the ProCom series have been designed to provide the information they need. This volume and the others in the series focus on what communication scholars have learned recently that might prove useful to professionals, how certain principles of interaction can be applied in concrete situations, and what difference the latest thoughts about communication can make in the lives and careers of professionals.

Most professionals want to improve their communication skills in the context of their unique professional callings. They don't want pie-in-the-sky solutions divorced from the reality of their jobs. And, because they are professionals, they typically distrust uninformed advice offered by uninformed advisors, no matter how well intentioned the advice and the advisors might be.

The books in this series have been carefully adapted to the needs and special circumstances of modern professionals. For example, it becomes obvious that the skills needed by a nurse when communicating with the family of a terminally ill patient will differ markedly from those demanded of an attorney when coaxing crucial testimony out of a reluctant witness. Furthermore, analyzing the nurse's or attorney's experiences will hardly help an engineer explain a new bridge's stress fractures to state legislators, a military officer motivate a group of especially dispirited recruits, or a police officer calm a vicious domestic disturbance. All these situations require a special kind of professional with a special kind of professional training. It is ProCom's intention to supplement that training in the area of communication skills.

Each of the authors of the ProCom volumes has extensively taught, written about, and listened to professionals in his or her area. In addition, the books have profited from the services of area consultants—working professionals who have practical experience with the special kinds of communication problems that confront their co-workers. The authors and the area consultants have collaborated to provide solutions to these vexing problems.

We, the editors of the series, believe that ProCom will treat you well. We believe that you will find no theory-for-the-sake-of-theory here. We believe that you will find a sense of expertise. We believe that you will find the content of the ProCom volumes to be specific rather than general, concrete rather than abstract, applied rather than theoretical. We believe that you will find the examples interesting, the information appropriate, and the applications useful. We believe that you will find the ProCom volumes helpful whether you read them on your own or use them in a workshop. We know that ProCom has brought together the most informed authors and the best analysis and advice possible. We ask you to add your own professional goals and practical experiences so that your human communication holds all the warmth that makes it human and all the clarity that makes it communication.

                                                Roderick P. Hart
                                                University of Texas at Austin

                                                Ronald L. Applbaum
                                                Pan American University

PREFACE

The Nurse's Guide to Better Communication has been written for nurses involved in primary nursing activities with patients or clients—it focuses on the communicative demands facing nurses in their day-to-day interactions with these patients or clients, with other nurses and health care professionals, and with all the other individuals involved in the health care process. The book is designed to be used by nurses individually, in continuing education workshops, and in nursing in-service programs. It can also be used as a supplemental text in a wide range of courses for student nurses.

The underlying premise of the book is that effective oral communication is a major determinant of effective nursing. Mastery of nursing knowledge, nursing skills, and communication skills are the key elements in successful nursing.

To help nurses become more effective communicators, oral communication theory is discussed as it applies to the individual nurse. This theory is presented in the context of information gained from interviews with working nurses. Practical exercises allow the reader to better understand her or his own communicative attitudes and behaviors and to implement sound communication principles in daily nursing practice.

The fundamental nursing communicative situation is identified as interaction between nurse and patient or client. Communication principles learned in conjunction with such two-party situations are expanded and applied to nonpatient/client two-party interactions, to interactions in which the nurse is a member of small groups and large organizations, and to nursing public speaking situations. Throughout the book, the nurse is encouraged to become an active participant through questions and exercises in order to develop personal principles and techniques that can be used in day-to-day nursing communicative situations.

To the many people who aided in the development of this book, thanks. Roderick Hart and Ronald Applbaum, the ProCom series editors, were stern taskmasters (in spite of what I may have said, I do appreciate your unbending ways). The reviewers, Nadine Littlefield, Dr. Fay L. Bower, Dr. Barbara Jackson, and Ruth Brooks, R.N., provided excellent suggestions and critiques. Roger Holloway, Anita Portugal, and the other staff at Scott, Foresman supplied direction, assistance, and kept the work on schedule. I don't have space to individually list all the nurses who provided interviews and suggestions, but thanks to all of you for "being the book."

To my wife and best friend, Mary Carlson, and to Margaret Kidwell Udin, thanks for being advisors, interviewers, and critics, providing emotional support, and teaching me what it means to be a nurse. To Ed and Greg, thanks for just being you.

Acknowledgments would not be complete without saying thanks to my colleagues in the Department of Communication at the University of Nebraska at Omaha who supplied encouragement and a conducive atmosphere to attempt this project, and to the University of Nebraska at Omaha Committee on Research which granted a summer fellowship that allowed research time for this book.

With the help of all these people, *The Nurse's Guide to Better Communication* is complete. However, the project will continue as long as nurses implement the guidelines and suggestions in these pages and in the process become more effective nurse communicators.

Robert E. Carlson

The Nurse's Guide to Better Communication

our opinion, that the professional status of nursing will dramatically increase simply by increasing educational requirements because there is a distinction between professional nurses and nurses as professionals. To remove some of the previously mentioned barriers requires *all* nurses be professional (whether the classification be L.P.N., A.D., Diploma, B.S.N., M.S.N. or vocational, technical, and professional).

NURSES AS PROFESSIONAL

What does it mean for all nurses to be professional? Nursing must provide technical skills for necessary "mechanical" medical services required for patient or client* well-being. Such services as taking patient temperatures and blood pressures, changing bandages, or even suctioning a tracheotomy are examples of "mechanical" services necessary for quality patient care. Nurses are essential for providing these services. However, quality patient care requires more from nursing.

Quality patient care requires that nurses possess vast nursing knowledge and possess something more. This "something more" is a major issue, in fact perhaps the major issue, for the professionalism of nursing. It is not obtained simply by educational degrees or years of educational training, although such formal learning can be a vehicle for this "extra."

What is it that makes a nurse a professional? No matter what rules and regulations are legislated concerning nursing licensure requirements, it is our position that, in addition to nursing knowledge and skills, nurses must possess a *specialized competence in communication*. For nurses to be successful, nurses must be able to communicate competently with patients, patients' family members, other nursing personnel, physicians and other health care team members, and with members of the general public.

Nurses need to be competent in communication. This statement should seem obvious to you and most, if not all of you, should readily agree. Intuitively, you know communication is important and each of you has been told countless times during nursing education and nursing practice that good communication is essential. "You must have good communication skills with clients." "The problem we have on this ward is communication." "We must better communicate with people in the support services." "I just can't communicate with that physician."

We can all agree on the need for good communication, but do we know what good communication is? Do we even know what communication is? Communication is similar to breathing—we breathe and communicate every day of our lives. If we are to survive, we must perform each

---

*For convenience, we will use the terms "patient" and "client" interchangeably throughout the book.

function with some degree of competence. As long as things are going satisfactorily we seldom think about our breathing or our communicating; it is only when there are problems do we consciously examine the processes involved.

Rather than just thinking about communication when problems exist, you must be sensitive to communication demands at all times during your nursing practice.

To be successful, it is a fairly safe generalization to state that all "professional" people need sound communicative techniques and skills. However, few if any professions place such complex communicative demands on their members than does nursing. A nurse is a person who is involved daily in crucial interpersonal contacts with patients and clients and must fulfill—constantly and simultaneously—the various roles of scientist, medical practitioner, human minister, and human being. In addition to confronting these patient/client demands, most nurses carry out their duties within a formal organizational structure such as a hospital, clinic, or educational institute.

Thus along with the interpersonal demands placed upon you in your interactions with patients, interpersonal demands are made of you by the organization in which you must function (nursing and non-nursing superiors, peers, and subordinates).

The crucial nature of daily nursing communicative demands is addressed by Barba Jean Edwards and John K. Brilhart, in the opening statement of their book *Communication in Nursing Practice* (1981): "Nursing communication skills, therapeutic or otherwise, are at the heart of all health care. They have gradually evolved into a major focus for nurses and other health care workers over the past few years." Also, Margaret L. Pluckhan in her 1978 book asserts:

> As I developed and wrote this manuscript, I was continuously questioning my boldness in entitling the book *Human Communication: The Matrix of Nursing*. I was going so far as to declare that communication was part of not only *most*, but *all* nursing functions. At this point I believe I have convinced myself of that fact, and I hope sufficient evidence has been presented to convince the reader as well.

A DEFINITION OF COMMUNICATION FOR NURSES

Before you can be sensitive to communication demands, you must understand what is involved in communication. Countless definitions and treatments of communication have been given in recent nursing literature. Many of the communication definitions are compatible with and typified by the following written by Mabel Hunsberger (1981):

> Communication is the sharing of information between individuals. Thoughts, feelings and opinions are exchanged, whether consciously or unconsciously, through verbal and nonverbal means. Relationships are formed through a continuous process of learning about what others think and feel. We are always communicating something, whether we are aware of it or not. The way messages are interpreted in the process of communication is dependent on the relationship that exists between the communicants.

While such definitions give you some insight into communication, they are incomplete and tell you little about how to be a more effective communicator. Let's examine the above definition in detail.

Communication does involve sharing, but it involves more—it involves creating. The sender of the message actively creates a message. All of the sender's attitudes, beliefs, values, previous experiences, and future expectations interact with the task at hand to form the basis for the message. This message is then transmitted to a receiver.

However, the message does not reach the receiver exactly as it left the sender. The environment surrounding the participants and the channel over which the message travels (that is, the direct link between the sender and the receiver) interact with the message to transform the message. In this transformation, the basic information content remains unchanged, however the value of the message changes. In a physical sense, the measurable amount of information in the message is the same when the message leaves the sender as when it reaches the receiver; however the usefulness and worth (that is, the value) of the information is very different to the sender or the receiver.

The transformation is not the end point of the communication process; it is only one step. Once the receiver has received the transformed message, the receiver applies her or his own attitudes, beliefs, values, previous experiences, and future expectations to this message. To describe this integration of message within the receiver, we shall use a term that has, in recent years, become the focus of many communication scholars. That term is *transaction*. The transaction forms the basis by which the receiver reacts and acts. In this process, the receiver becomes the sender and the cycle repeats itself.

It is important to point out that, although the process of communication we have described is cyclical in which the information output of one person becomes the input for the other person, the process is not a simple stimulus-response phenomenon. Stimulus-response is involved but because of the transformations and transactions occurring, something new is created that is more than the individual's thoughts, feelings, and opinions.

To further complicate the communicative picture, these processes are happening on conscious and subconscious levels and through spoken (verbal) and nonspoken (nonverbal) means. Many nonverbal communication experts estimate that in a normal two-party interaction, only one-third of the social meaning is obtained through verbal components; two-thirds of the meaning is derived through the nonverbal aspects.

Our conscious and/or subconscious are always acting and reacting in a two-party interaction and because of this, a phrase that has become a cliché in communication literature over the past decade, can be stated an indisputable fact. That phrase articulated in 1967 by Paul Watzlawick, Janet Beavin, and Don Jackson is: YOU CANNOT NOT COMMUNICATE.

When two people are in each other's presence in any manner (face to face or even just linked by a telephone system) communication is always and continuously taking place. And each of these communicative events has direct and unerasable impact on any future interactions between the individuals involved. Relationships formed not only contribute to message interpretation but also, message interpretation contributes to relationship formation.

What then is communication? In our view, *communication is a dynamic process in which information is consciously and subconsciously created by a person, transmitted and transformed through verbal and nonverbal methods and recreated in a transactional manner by a receiver. This process continues in an evolving manner in which relationships are defined and developed and in turn define and develop subsequent communicative activities.*

What implications does it have for you as to how you define communication? If you define communication as simply a process of sharing or exchange, you can gain some insight into understanding some of the individual components involved in communication, but you can develop few practical guidelines that will aid you in day-to-day nursing communicative encounters. However, if you expand your definition to include the individual creative dynamics involved in communicative processes, then perhaps you will be able to develop qualities that will result in more successful interpersonal communicative experiences.

The task for you in the remainder of this book is to understand what this definition of communication means; to learn basic communicative principles and techniques; and to integrate the ideas presented within yourself to better facilitate effective nursing communication.

Because of inherent uncertainties in any individual's creative processes, we offer no lists of "always do this; never do that." We offer no guarantees; all we offer is generalized guidelines that require constant work if you hope to become a more competent communicator.

The Range of Nursing Oral Communicative Demands

What was discussed so far in terms of communication has involved only two people interacting. One of the major reasons for starting at this point is our belief that the primary focus of nursing is two-party communicative situations involving a nurse and an other—that other being a patient, a patient family member, another nurse, a physician, another health care team member, etc.

However, two-party communicative situations are not the only communicative situations in which you are involved. Communicative demands are also placed upon you in small groups (which we will define as 3 to 12 people), organizational settings (involving more than 12 people), and public speaking situations (in which you must address a large group of people). Each of these communicative situations (or "configurations" as they are often called) places unique demands upon you. However, we shall attempt to show how the generalized guidelines we develop when discussing two-party nursing communication can be expanded and applied to each of these other communicative settings.

What has been stated so far about communication can be applied to any profession. Before giving specifics concerning nursing communication, we must ask, how is nursing communication special from other professions' communicative demands and why is communicative competency so critical for nurses?

THE ROLE OF NURSING AND COMMUNICATION

One way that we can gain some insight into the uniqueness of nursing communication is to examine the nature of the nursing role and how this role has changed over the past several years.

We conducted in-depth interviews with approximately forty nurses from a variety of health care organizations in several states, who were representative of the present educational levels of nursing, and who worked in a wide range of specialities within nursing. We did not randomly select nurse interviewees, but rather selected our interviewees because they were recognized by other nurses as being technically competent and particularly successful communicators (although, during our selection process, no attempt was made to define for anyone what we meant by "successful communication").

DISCUSSION QUESTION

The first questions we asked our nurse respondents, and we ask of you are: "What is your perception of the role of the nurse? Has that perception changed since you first entered nursing?"

Typical responses received to these questions are given below. Responses are *verbatim quotes* made from tape recordings of the interviews. The interviewer in each interview was one of the two nursing area consultants and is designated by "R"; the interviewee was a nurse respondent and is designated by "E."

E is a diploma graduate, twenty years experience, primary area is coronary care, presently in a nursing administrative position.

R. What is your perception of the role of a nurse? Has that perception changed since you started working? If so, how?

E. In the twenty years of nursing I do feel that the role of a nurse has changed tremendously and I believe it has changed for the better. In nursing twenty years ago an RN worked mainly with the patient—hands-on type care. They did bed baths, enemas, general things for the patient. This has changed over the years. We have included licensed practical nurses and nurse aides to do the majority of the hands-on care—RNs have picked up a teaching role. We have gone to preventive health care. The nurses work with the patients in teaching them about their disease or their illness as a preventive type thing and also so that they can have a better perception of what they are doing when they go home. Twenty years ago, we always told the patient if they asked what medicine they were on or what their blood pressure was or anything in this line, we couldn't tell them. The doctor ordered the medicine so you are supposed to take it, or your blood pressure will be recorded and your doctor will talk to you about it. This type thing. Now we may tell all the patients whatever information they want, being it blood pressures or medicines. If they ask what the medicine is, they have the option of not taking it if they don't want to take it. They must know what it is and the side effects and really what to look for and what it is going to do for them. So I do think that the role of the nurse has changed and it has gone to more of a teaching professional type nurse.

E is an A.D. graduate, four years experience, primary area is extended care.

R. What is your perception of the role of a nurse?

E. Well, I believe my biggest responsibility is helping people in the health care situation get through their illness phase, rehabilitation, and preventative teaching. I view as one of my primary responsibilities to prevent recurrence of those existing health problems.

R. Has that perception changed since you started working?

The Role of Nursing and Communication 9

E. I find it difficult a lot of times to fulfill all of the goals that I had set while I was a student. But I keep those goals in mind to kind of help me through the difficult working situation. A lot of times we just don't have time to fulfill completely all of these goals.

E is a B.S.N. graduate, eight years experience, primary area is working with handicapped and retarded patients.

R. What is your perception of the role of a nurse?

E. My perception of the role of a nurse is that she or he works with the client to foster and provide health maintenance. The nurse also fosters health with the family and in the community.

R. Could you define client?

E. It can be a patient in the hospital or a person outside the hospital. It can be somebody who is acutely or chronically ill or in need.

R. Has that perception changed since you started working?

E. It has changed. Because when I began working with handicapped and retarded clients, I thought that the nurse was an advocate who took over the role of the family. Now I see the family system as usually a pretty functional system and I see the nurse's role as primarily assisting that system, not substituting for it.

E is a diploma graduate, six years experience, primary area is community health.

R. What is your perception of your role as a nurse?

E. As someone to work with the doctor in helping to implement patient care. I guess most nurses feel they are not handmaidens to the doctor to carry out every whim that he says. I think that we really have a responsibility to question and help the doctor work with patients in the home or in the hospital. Because we spend more time with the patient, and a lot of times I think nurses pick up things that doctors don't even see, so we really have to work with the doctor as far as helping him with diagnosis and treatment plan. For example, if the patient had an ulcer or a bedsore and it wasn't healing properly, the nurse would be the one to inform the doctor of this and bring it to his attention, because if the nurse didn't say this then he would just assume that everything was going well. I think even more so in the home when the nurse is visiting. The doctor usually doesn't get a chance to visit the client as often or to spend the time like the nurse does or to know the stress factors in the home and the other things working within the family.

R. In your perception of the role of the nurse, have your perceptions changed since you started working? And, if so, how?

E. I think they have. I think especially working with community health I was out to cure the world when I first started and in some respect I still like to believe this but I think I now look at it as a more realistic thing than idealistic. I've learned that you care for patients on their level and the patient is the one in charge, not you. You should be working to meet their needs and not your needs. It's not something that you force on the patient—it is something that the patient should want to see too. I don't think that you get very far just working with your needs if you don't help with what they have to offer and with what they want also.

E is a recent B.S.N. graduate, nine years experience as an aide and operating room technician; primary area is medical/surgical.

R. What is your perception of the role of a nurse?

E. It's someone that's there to help the patient and be able to communicate to the doctor the progress that the patient has so that he can be able to treat the patient.

R. Has your perception changed since you started working?

E. Well, it has changed since I started in the medical field nine years ago but it's just since I've been in nursing school that my opinion has become a strong personal belief. The nurse is there to help more than to be a servant.

R. When you first began nine years ago, you saw the nurse as a servant to the doctor?

E. Yes.

R. And now that's changing through your education?

E. Yes.

E is a diploma and B.S.N. graduate, nine years experience, primary area is newborn ICU.

R. What is your perception of the role of a nurse?

E. I can't answer that in one sentence.
It depends on the situation—the nurse has to perform many roles.

R. Has your perception changed since you started working?

E. Yes.

R. How has it changed?

E. When I first started working I thought the nurse should provide only technical skills. Now I think the nurse must be able to not only deal with technical aspects of health care but many other areas such as emotional needs of families.

E is an A.D. graduate, eleven years experience, primary area is operating room.

R. What is your perception of the role of a nurse?

E. You mean how I see what the role of a nurse is?

R. Yes.

E. Day-to-day care; primary nursing care of a patient. Total care of the patient.

R. How has this perception changed since you started working? And how?

E. It hasn't changed in my personal job in the O.R. but it has changed for patient care on the hospital wards—on the ward much more is required of the nurse than it used to be.

E is a B.S.N., M.S.N., 29 years experience, primary area is nursing education.

R. What is your perception of the role of a nurse?

E. My perception is that the role of a nurse is multifaceted. Speaking broadly, the nurse is an educator, a researcher, a person who devotes time for community service. More specifically, the nurse is a person involved in leadership roles, communication processes, and all the processes in which nurses deal and that would include decision maker and change maker. So I believe that it is multifaceted—it's not the limited role of the traditional bedside nurse. I don't want to say bedside nursing is unimportant because it is extremely important. But I think nurses do all the things I mentioned before in addition to giving bedside care. I think now the role of the nurse has expanded to more family and community problems. The nurse practices more of her or his roles in other environments and other situations rather than just acute care settings.

R. Has that perception of nursing changed since you started working?

E. No, I can't really say that it has. My personal perception is the same, but I think this expanded, multifaceted role is being recognized and adopted more and more.

From our interviews several major issues stand out. There is no one role of the nurse. Rather there are many roles that are continually in flux—changing for the individual nurse and changing for the profession of nursing. Nurses are becoming increasingly involved not only in providing bedside care but also in providing preventive health care services through teaching clients, clients' families, and other health care professionals. Nurses are receiving and accepting more responsibilities in terms of health care delivery. Nurses are providing more emotional support services for clients, taking more responsibility for physical assessments, providing more constructive information to physicians, and serving as the vital link as patient advocate in the health care system. Finally, nurses are taking on more and more leadership roles in a wide variety of health care settings and situations. How many of these issues did you mention in your responses?

There is one key that is essential in all these areas for nurses to be successful—that key is effective communication. Few professions place such complex role and associated communicative demands upon their members. Nursing is evolving into a profession based upon communication—communication, in our opinion, is becoming the very essence of nursing. It is not sufficient for a nurse to possess medical and technical knowledge and skills. The nurse, to be successful, must also be communicatively competent. *Effective nursing embodies nursing knowledge, nursing skills, and effective communication.*

NURSING COMMUNICATIVE COMPETENCE

A person is unlikely to complete requirements for a nursing degree, unlikely to pass state board examinations, and even more unlikely to maintain a nursing job, if she or he lacks nursing skill or knowledge. But what about communication competence? What has nursing done to ensure communication competence?

DISCUSSION QUESTION

What training have you had in communication?

From our experience and the experience of our nurse respondents, it appears that while nursing recognizes the importance of communication, relatively little has been done to develop communication competence in individual nurses.

In the course of our interviews, most A.D. graduates reported, at most, two weeks of formal training in communication during their nursing degree program; diploma and B.S.N. graduates typically reported having some communication training in psychology courses, and B.S.N. graduates also reported having a basic public speaking or interpersonal communication course. A few of our respondents reported having taken an advanced communication class such as group discussion or interviewing but these were usually taken as elective courses. Many of our respondents, regardless of the nursing degree, had attended at least one workshop or nursing in-service devoted to communication. However, an almost universal response we obtained during the interviews went like this:

My communication training has been done mostly by myself on the job. I have learned through trial and error what communication techniques will work and what will not work in certain types of situations. I know what is likely to work, but I don't know why it works.

How can nurses obtain effective communication skills? While formal courses, workshops, in-services, and even books concerning communication can all aid in developing communication competence, they are not sufficient no matter how many are employed to ensure communication competence. Skill in communication can be obtained only through hard work on your part. If you follow our suggestions, we cannot guarantee you will become a "perfect" communicator, but if you think about these suggestions and continually work at communication, chances are that you will be a successful communicator.

We are now in a position to ask the specific question: "What is effective nursing communication?" At the risk of disappointing those who desire a direct, simple answer, we will answer by saying: "It depends." Effective communication depends on your goals, your knowledge, your entire being; it depends on the other's goals, knowledge, and being; it depends on the specific situation. Since there are so many contingencies, all that we can do in this book is to help you gain insight into some of those "it depends."

COMMUNICATIVE ATTITUDE SETS

In accord with our earlier conceptualization of communication, we will first discuss YOU in terms of your internal communicative generating process. It was stated that you apply your attitudes, beliefs, values, previous experiences, and future expectations to the communicative task at hand to form the basis for the message you will send.

Many attempts have been made to distinguish attitudes from beliefs from values from opinions, etc. However, an adequate distinction has not been formulated primarily because of the interrelated nature of all these concepts. Rather than try to distinguish these bits of our internal make-up, we would rather look at them as a whole in their relation to the communication generating process. We shall call this whole *attitudes toward encoding messages*. Encoding means what occurs within your mind immediately before you verbally (or nonverbally) say something. Sets of your encoding attitudes have interwoven within them your beliefs, values, and prior experiences.

Your author along with Roderick P. Hart of the University of Texas at Austin and William F. Eadie of California State University-Northridge developed a self-report measuring instrument for assessing attitude sets toward encoding messages called the RHETSEN instrument.

The RHETSEN Instrument

Listed below are a number of statements. Respond to each statement individually and indicate your opinion by marking one of the following in Column 1 (Columns 2; 3a and b; and 4a and b will be used at a later time to score the questionnaire):

A=almost always true; **B**=frequently true; **C**=sometimes true; **D**=infrequently true; **E**=almost never true

	Column 1 (your response)	Column 2	Column 3		Column 4	
			a	b	a	b

1. People should be frank and spontaneous in conversation.
2. An idea can be communicated in many different ways.
3. When talking with someone with whom you disagree, you should feel obligated to state your opinion.
4. A person should laugh at an unfunny joke just to please the joke-teller.
5. It's good to follow the rule: before blowing your top at someone, sleep on the problem.
6. When talking to others, you should drop all of your defenses.
7. It is best to hide one's true feelings in order to avoid hurting others.
8. No matter how hard you try, you just can't make friends with everyone.
9. One should keep quiet rather than say something which will alienate others.
10. You should share your joys with your friends.
11. It is acceptable to discuss religion with a stranger.
12. A supervisor in a work situation must be forceful with subordinates to be effective.
13. A person should tell it like it is.
14. "Look before you leap" is the most important rule to follow when talking to others.
15. You should tell friends if you think they are making a mistake.
16. The first thing that comes to mind is the best thing to say.
17. When conversing, you should tell others what they want to hear.
18. When someone dominates the conversation, it's important to interrupt that person in order to state your opinion.

	Column 1 (your response)	Column 2	Column 3 a	Column 3 b	Column 4 a	Column 4 b

19. When angry, a person should say nothing rather than say something he or she will be sorry for later.
20. When someone has an irritating habit, he or she should be told about it.
21. When talking to your friends, you should adjust your remarks to suit them.
22. You really can't put sugar coating on bad news.
23. A person who speaks his or her gut feelings is to be admired.
24. You shouldn't make a scene in a restaurant by arguing with a waiter.
25. Putting thoughts into words just the way you want them is a difficult process.
26. A friend who has bad breath should be told about it.
27. If you're sure you're right, you should argue with a person who disagrees with you.
28. If people would open up to each other the world would be better off.
29. There is a difference between someone who is "diplomatic" and one who is "two-faced."
30. You should tell people if you think they are about to embarrass themselves.
31. One should not be afraid to voice his or her opinion.
32. If your boss doesn't like you, there's not much you can do about it.
33. You should tell someone if you think he or she is giving you bad advice.
34. Saying what you think is a sign of friendship.
35. When you're sure you're right, you should press your point until you win the argument.
36. "If you feel it, say it" is a good rule to follow in conversation.
37. If a man cheats on his wife, he should tell her.
38. It is better to speak your gut feelings than to beat around the bush.
39. We should have a kind word for the people we meet in life.
40. One should treat all people in the same way.

The Nurse as Communicator

The RHETSEN instrument is contained on pages 14 and 15. Following the instrument are scoring procedures, a discussion of what these scores mean, and normative data obtained from nurses involved in a variety of nursing settings and situations.

You are asked to complete the questionnaire *before* reading the discussion. Your individual responses to the questionnaire will give you a measure of your internal attitudes toward communication—attitudinal sets of which you may or may not be consciously aware. But by becoming aware, hopefully you will be able to use the ideas contained in the remaining pages and build upon your internal make-up to become a more competent and successful communicator.

There are no absolutely "right" or "wrong" answers to the questions. For the instrument to be of value, you must answer the questions honestly.

Scoring Instructions for RHETSEN

In Column 2 for the following items, mark 2 if your answer in Column 1 is C; mark 1 if your answer in Column 1 is B or D; and mark 0 if your answer in Column 1 is A or E: Items: 1, 3, 4, 5, 7, 9, 11, 13, 15, 16, 17, 18, 19, 20, 21, 23, 24, 26, 27, 28, 30, 31, 33, 34, 35, 37, 38, 39.

Add the total numbers you marked in Column 2 and place this total at the bottom of Column 2. Totals can range from 0 to 56.

In Column 3a for the following items, mark 2 if your answer in Column 1 is A; mark 1 if your answer in Column 1 is B; and mark 0 if your answer in Column 1 is C, D, or E: Items: 1, 3, 11, 13, 15, 16, 18, 20, 23, 26, 27, 28, 30, 31, 33, 34, 35, 38.

In Column 3b for the following items, mark 2 if your answer in Column 1 is E; mark 1 if your answer in Column 1 is D; and mark 0 if your answer in Column 1 is A, B, or C: Items: 4, 5, 7, 9, 17, 21.

Add the total numbers you marked in Columns 3a *and* 3b and place this total at the bottom of Column 3. Totals can range from 0 to 48.

In Column 4a for the following items, mark 2 if your answer in Column 1 is E; mark 1 if your answer in Column 1 is D; and mark 0 if your answer in Column 1 is A, B, or C: Items: 1, 3, 12, 13, 15, 16, 18, 20, 23, 26, 27, 28, 30, 33, 34, 35, 38.

In Column 4b for the following items, mark 2 if your answer in Column 1 is A; mark 1 if your answer in Column 1 is B; and mark 0 if your answer in Column 1 is C, D, or E: Items: 4, 5, 7, 9, 17, 19, 24.

Add the total numbers you marked in Columns 4a *and* 4b and place this total at the bottom of Column 4. Totals can range from 0 to 48.

Interpretation of RHETSEN Scores

The number total in Column 2 is your Rhetorical Sensitivity (RS) score; Column 3 contains your Noble Self (NS) score; and Column 4 contains your Rhetorical Reflector (RR) score. Each of these scores is a measure of your adherence to a particular communicative attitude set. The three attitude sets (RS, NS, RR) are not the only attitude sets that you could embrace, however they are the three major "pure" orientations, and taken together define potential attitude sets.

Very few individuals completely embrace any one of the pure sets—most of us function in accord with degrees of each of the pure sets. When your three scores are considered as a whole, a profile emerges which describes your internal communicative orientation.

Before we can discuss what your individual scores mean for you as a nurse, we must first briefly describe what each of these three attitudinal sets mean in their generalized form.

Rhetorical Sensitivity. Among the characteristics of a person who aligns herself or himself with the Rhetorical Sensitivity construct are the following: This person believes that seldom if ever should a person say the first thing that comes to mind in a frank and spontaneous manner—the implications and consequences of expressing our initial reactions must be considered.

Such a person also recognizes that there is a difference between an idea and the way in which that idea can be expressed—any idea can be expressed in a multitude of ways. Not only does this person recognize the multiplicity of ways of expressing ideas, but also is willing to search through the various alternatives and select and enact the best alternative for the self, the other, and the situation. In this process, the primary goal is not just to serve the needs of the self or not just to serve the needs of the other but rather to serve the needs of both self and other within the constraints of the particular situation.

A Rhetorically Sensitive person is constantly weighing the potential consequences of communicative choices and attempting to enact the best possible alternative for the other and the situation all the while maintaining one's own self-interests and integrity.

Noble Self. A Noble Self, on the other hand, believes that one must be frank, open, and totally honest in expressing one's feelings. The self is the overriding concern. Self is a consistent, unified, and a singular concept. Successful communication from such a perspective is achieved when the self is expressed and the needs of the self are fulfilled—the needs of the other and situational demands are unimportant.

Noble Selves expect others to also be consistent, unified, and open about their feelings, desires, etc. In interactions with others, a Noble

Self's goal is to achieve and maintain control. This control is over oneself, over the other, and over the situation. To compromise from such a position is a sign of weakness. The Noble Self position was popularized in the 1960s and early 1970s and was expressed by such phrases as: "Look out for number one" and "Be true to yourself."

Rhetorical Reflector. A third major alternative attitude set is that of the Rhetorical Reflector. For a Rhetorical Reflector, the overriding concern is serving the wants and desires of others. Rhetorical Reflectors perceive of no real self to call their own—their goal in communication is to attempt to discover what will please the other and to carry out the other's wishes.

The Rhetorical Reflector desires no control over others, situations, and even over herself or himself. The other guides communicative events. The life of a Rhetorical Reflector is one of service and obeying the dictates of others. It does not matter for a Rhetorical Reflector how much she or he is inconvenienced or suffers, as long as the other is satisfied and pleased.

Formation and Implications to Nursing of Communicative Attitude Sets

We have just highlighted the three constructs—Rhetorical Sensitivity, Noble Self, and Rhetorical Reflector. Few, if any, of us embody 100 percent of the behaviors of the three constructs, but most of us embrace various aspects of each.

Many contributing factors merge to formulate our exact positions. Our research has shown that a wide variety of demographic, cultural, and social factors merge to influence individual communicative attitudinal orientations. (See, for example, Hart, Carlson, and Eadie, 1980; and Carlson, 1978, 1980.) Factors such as age, sex, ethnic background, formal education, socioeconomic class, religious and political orientations, geographic location of residence, size of family, and marital status all directly relate to our attitude formation. In part because of all of these factors, we cannot state that any particular RHETSEN scores are good or bad. However, we can make the statement that *most nurses can be more effective communicators if they increase their level of Rhetorical Sensitivity.*

Research that your author conducted in 1978 involving advanced level nursing students provides support for the statement advocating an increase in your level of Rhetorical Sensitivity. Students were asked to complete the RHETSEN scale and their nursing instructors, unaware of their students' results, were asked to rate all of their students on various nursing dimensions.

The following were among the results that were obtained. The more Rhetorically Sensitive the student as indicated by RS score:

- the higher the student was rated as providing quality nursing care
- the better the student performed on written classroom examinations which tested principles of quality nursing care implementation
- the better the student was perceived as communicating with patients in routine nursing situations
- the better the student was perceived as communicating with patients in crisis situations
- the better the student was perceived as communicating with peers
- the less nervous the student was perceived when interacting with nursing role superiors

Concomitantly, the more Noble Self and/or Rhetorical Reflector as indicated by NS and RR score respectively, the more opposite the student was perceived on all of the above dimensions. Of particular note was the result that the higher the student's level of Noble Self, the worse the student was rated in terms of providing quality nursing care and performing on written examinations. Also, the higher the Rhetorical Reflector score, the more nervous the student was perceived when interacting with superiors. High levels of Noble Self and/or high levels of Rhetorical Reflector were found to be approximately equally associated with poor ratings in ability to communicate with patients in routine and in crisis situations.

While we have not obtained performance ratings of working nurses and correlated these with RHETSEN scores, we have amassed data relating RHETSEN scores to many self-reported data from working nurses.

Data obtained from 1977 to 1982 during research involving hundreds of nurses throughout the country, representing all present levels of nursing, and a wide variety of nursing areas and organizations, allows us to present some normative data to which you can compare yourself. From this data, *we do not want you to conclude that you are a good or bad nurse or make any other judgments.* At this point, you should simply understand what your communicative attitude set is in relation to other nurses.

On the RS scale, most of you will score between 25 and 37; on the NS scale between 7 and 19; and on the RR scale between 3 and 13.

The three individual scales were not constructed in exactly the same manner, so the magnitudes of the ranges are not comparable to each other. Thus, if you had a score of 32 on the RS scale, 16 on the NS scale,

FIGURE 1 RHETSEN Mean Scores According to Professional Nurses' Reported Actual Work Areas

Rhetorical Sensitivity Scale		Noble Self Scale		Rhetorical Reflector Scale	
Area	Mean (average) Score	Area	Mean (average) Score	Area	Mean (average) Score
Rehabilitation	37.8	Ambulance	21.8	Extended Care	12.9
Outpatient	37.0	Urology/Cardiology	16.3	Newborn Intensive Care	10.0
Newborn Intensive Care	34.0	Supervision	16.2	Medical/Surgical	8.9
Psychiatric	32.0	Orthopedics	15.3	Maternity/Newborn	8.9
Medical/Surgical	31.0	Operating Room	14.8	Operating Room	8.8
Intensive Care/Recovery	30.6	Multiple Areas	14.6	Intensive Care/Recovery	8.6
Emergency Room	30.5	Psychiatric	13.6	Emergency Room	8.6
Maternity/Newborn	30.4	Intensive Care/Recovery	13.1	Orthopedics	8.5
Pediatrics	30.3	Pediatrics	12.9	Urology/Cardiology	8.3
Multiple Areas	29.9	Maternity/Newborn	12.8	Supervision	8.2
Operating Room	28.5	Emergency Room	12.8	Pediatrics	7.9
Orthopedics	28.2	Medical/Surgical	12.4	Multiple Areas	7.7
Urology/Cardiology	27.8	Rehabilitation	11.8	Ambulance	6.8
Supervision	27.7	Extended Care	11.4	Outpatient	6.0
Extended Care	26.9	Newborn Intensive Care	9.4	Psychiatric	5.9
Ambulance	24.3	Outpatient	8.9	Rehabilitation	2.8

and 8 on the RR scale, you could not say that you were twice as Rhetorically Sensitive as Rhetorical Reflector and twice as Noble Self as Rhetorical Reflector. Each scale score must be interpreted separately. Use the ranges given to compare yourself to other nurses on each individual scale.

As mentioned earlier, many demographic, cultural, and social factors all influence your individual scores. In addition, from data obtained from working nurses, we can also state the following specifics about nurses' RHETSEN scores. The older you are, the more likely your RS score will be in the low range and the RR score in the high range. In general, the more formal schooling you have had, especially in terms of communication training, the higher will be your RS score and the lower your NS and RR scores.

We have also discovered that nursing job and organizational demands may be related to specific attitudinal orientations. As an example of the data suggesting these potential nursing duty influences, Figure 1 lists mean scores (average scores) on the three scales (RS, NS, RR) obtained from a survey of 537 nursing personnel who worked in three Indiana hospitals. The areas listed are the hospital areas in which the respondents reported they worked and may differ in terms of organization and function from areas in hospitals in which many of you work or are familiar.

Because of many uncontrolled variables, conclusions from the data must be made cautiously. However, one conclusion that can be made from this data and other data we have obtained is that some areas of nursing either foster and/or attract nurses with certain types of attitudinal sets. Based upon our knowledge of the hospitals and other organizational units surveyed, and the structure, functions, and duties of the particular areas within these organizational settings, it appears that nurses in areas in which their main job involves communication, score highest on the RS scale and lowest on the NS and RR scales. Next highest on the RS scale were nurses whose primary jobs involved communication with infants, children, and client's family members; and also nurses who occasionally were in high stress situations. These two groups of nurses also scored relatively low on the NS scale and moderately high on the RR scale. Nurses who were primarily involved in high stress situations or nurses whose main job involved nonpatient communication scored lowest on the RS scale, highest on the NS scale, and had moderately high RR scores.

NURSING PROFESSIONALISM AND RHETORICAL SENSITIVITY

One additional result from our RHETSEN research that must be mentioned is the following: When nursing students' and actual nurses' RHETSEN scores are compared to the scores of students and graduates in other fields who have comparable demographic, social, and cultural backgrounds, nursing students and nurses generally score lower on the RS scale and higher on the RR scale than comparison groups. We have obtained some recent data that these discrepancies are becoming less but there still are significant differences.

What do these results mean for nursing? Returning to the issues that began this chapter, one possible interpretation is that nurses have in the past perceived themselves and have developed communicative attitudes in such a manner that their primary goals were to please and to serve others.

While we do not want to condemn such a stance, in our opinion, if nurses desire to be recognized as true professionals, they as a group must develop more flexible attitudes in which they are still "providers" but yet maintain their own self-integrity. *In other words, it is our opinion that professionalism of nursing depends in part on nurses as a group becoming more Rhetorically Sensitive.*

While it cannot be stated that simply holding Rhetorically Sensitive attitudes will result in communication competence, our research results seem to overwhelmingly suggest that the chances of being communicatively competent dramatically increase when levels of Rhetorical Sensitivity increase.

Does this mean that we recommend all nurses be totally Rhetorically Sensitive? By no means, for many nursing situations, such as situations that involve life and death issues, dictate that nurses cannot always carefully weigh the interpersonal consequences of communicative actions. Sometimes the nurse must rely on professional judgment and dictate communicative outcomes; at times, the nurse must enact characteristics of a Noble Self.

Likewise, certain nursing situations call for total giving of self and meeting the demands of the other. In certain situations, the proper nursing response is simply to follow orders or to serve the needs of others; at times, the nurse must enact characteristics of a Rhetorical Reflector.

Depending on type of nursing, kinds of patients/clients and organizational structure, nurses, if they are to be effective, will, to varying degrees, be required to be Noble Selves and/or Rhetorical Reflectors. However, few if any nurses can hope to be communicatively and professionally effective if they constantly and continuously embrace attitudes of the Noble Self or Rhetorical Reflector.

To restate, it is only by being Rhetorically Sensitive do we believe that nurses as a group can be effective communicators and professional. If nurses do embrace Rhetorical Sensitivity, inherently they will also have at their disposal the orientation to enact other attitudinal sets if necessary.

The question facing us is how specifically can you as a nurse become more Rhetorically Sensitive when you are a member of a small chapters. We shall begin by detailing what it takes, in our opinion, for you to become more Rhetorically Sensitive in one-to-one situations. Theory, basic definitions, and principles of one-to-one communication will be presented, and you will be asked to apply this knowledge to specific situations involving a nurse and a patient/client. Next, we shall discuss communication-related principles to include one-to-one situations in which a nurse interacts with nonpatients/clients. Then our basic principles will be carried over and expanded in an attempt to help you become more Rhetorically Sensitive when you are a member of a small group, a large organization, or involved in public (one-to-many) communication.

SUMMARY

In this chapter we have asserted nursing's need to develop professionalism in all its members. This professionalism involves both nursing skill competence and communicative competence. Communication is defined as a dynamic process in which information is consciously and subconsciously created by a person, transmitted and transformed through verbal and nonverbal methods, and recreated in a transactional manner by a receiver. In light of the rapidly expanding role of nursing, we have stressed the increasing importance of effective communication by nurses.

To help you develop your communication competence, you examined your communicative attitudes as measured by the RHETSEN instrument. Comparative data obtained from extensive research involving nurses was supplied to help you understand your own communicative orientation. Based upon our research, we advocate each of you, as a nurse, increase your level of Rhetorical Sensitivity if you desire to become a more effective nursing communicator.

To increase Rhetorical Sensitivity means that you must develop attitudes in which you more carefully consider the range of communicative options available to you in any particular interpersonal situation; that you weigh the consequences of enacting each option; and that you select and enact the option that best serves the needs of others and the situation, all the while however, maintaining your own self-integrity.

Our task in the remaining chapters can be stated simply: *How do you as nurses develop and implement Rhetorical Sensitivity in your day-to-day professional contacts?*

References

Carlson, R. E. Rhetorical sensitivity: theoretical perspective, measurement, and implications in an interpersonal and organizational context (Doctoral dissertation, Purdue University, 1978). *Dissertation Abstracts International,* 1978, *39,* 2615A. (University Microfilms No. 78-21, 426).

Carlson, R. E. *Rhetorical sensitivity and the nursing profession.* Paper presented at the annual convention of the Central States Speech Association, Chicago, Illinois, April 1980.

Critical care nurses support baccalaureate. *The American Nurse,* 1982, 14, No. 4, p. 10.

Edwards, B. J., & Brilhart, J. K. *Communication in nursing practice.* St. Louis, MO: The C. V. Mosby Company, 1981, p. v.

Hart, R. P., Carlson, R. E., & Eadie, W. F. Attitudes toward communication and the assessment of rhetorical sensitivity. *Communication Monographs,* 1980, *47,* 1-22.

Hunsberger, M. Communicating with children. In J. J. M. Tackett & M. Hunsberger (Eds.), *Family-centered care of children and adolescents.* Philadelphia: W. B. Saunders Company, 1981, p. 166.

NLN endorses baccalaureate for entry. *The American Nurse,* 1982, 14, No. 4, pp. 3; 10.

Photo section featuring nurses cancelled by *Playboy* magazine. *The American Nurse*, 1982, 14, No. 4, p. 32.

Participants at entry into practice meeting agree on baccalaureate; disagree on terminology. *American Journal of Nursing*, 1978, 78, No. 4, pp. 535; 560; 562; 565.

Pluckhan, M. L. *Human communication: The matrix of nursing*. New York: McGraw-Hill Book Company, 1978, p. 136.

Watzlawick, P., Beavin, J. H., & Jackson, D. D. *Pragmatics of human communication*. New York: W. W. Norton & Co., Inc., 1967.

Suggested Readings

Interpersonal Communication

Crable, R. E. *One to another: A guidebook for interpersonal communication*. New York: Harper & Row, Publishers, 1981.
An easy to read and theoretically sound introduction into the nature of human communication and fundamentals concerning interpersonal communication. An excellent starting point for readers unfamiliar with interpersonal communication theory.

Smith, D. R., & Williamson, L. K. *Interpersonal communication: Roles, rules, strategies, and games* (2nd ed.). Dubuque, Iowa: Wm. C. Brown Company Publishers, 1981.
An advanced level exploration of interpersonal communication. Designed for readers already having some familiarity with interpersonal communication theory. Places great emphasis on the transactional nature of human communication.

Nursing Communication

Edwards, B. J., & Brilhart, J. K. *Communication in nursing practice*. St. Louis, MO: The C. V. Mosby Company, 1981.
A broad in scope textbook approach to oral communication principles and practices as applied to nursing. Well grounded in communication theory and interspersed with real life nursing examples.

Pluckhan, M. L. *Human communication: The matrix of nursing*. New York: McGraw-Hill Book Company, 1978.
An excellent theoretical discussion of oral communication. A limited attempt to implement communication theory into nursing practice.

Rhetorical Sensitivity

Darnell, D. K., & Brockriede, W. *Persons communicating*. Englewood Cliffs, NJ: Prentice-Hall, Inc., 1976.
Provides an overview of the rhetorical approach to human communication. Introduces the concepts of Noble Self and Rhetorical Reflector.

Hart, R. P., & Burks, D. M. Rhetorical sensitivity and social interaction. *Speech Monographs,* 1972, *39,* 75-91.
   The first articulation of Rhetorical Sensitivity. A theoretical presentation of the rhetorical perspective toward human communication.

Hart, R. P., Carlson, R. E., & Eadie, W. F. Attitudes toward communication and the assessment of rhetorical sensitivity. *Communication Monographs,* 1980, *47,* 1-22.
   Expansion and application of the concepts introduced by Hart and Burks and by Darnell and Brockriede. Describes the development of the RHETSEN instrument, and reports extensive research findings obtained through use of the instrument.

CHAPTER 2

The Nurse as Interviewer

Of all the communication demands placed on the nurse, the most important communicative function often takes place in one-to-one situations. We shall label such one-to-one interactions *interviews*. Our use of the word "interview" may be different from the definition to which you are accustomed. We use the word for very specific reasons which shall be explained.

A DEFINITION OF AN INTERVIEW

Our definition of an interview will be a slight modification of a definition given by communication experts Robert Goyer, W. Charles Redding, and John Rickey (1968). We shall define an interview as: two people, at least one of whom has a distinct purpose in reference to the other, and both of whom speak and listen from time to time. Let's examine what this definition means in a nursing context.

Two People

While group interviews are possible, we want to restrict ourselves for the present to situations that involve only two people—nurse and patient, nurse and physician, nurse and another nurse, etc. Such two-party interactions are the most common and, in our opinion, the most important communicative configurations confronting a nurse. Not only are such situations critical to the role of nursing but they are also the context in which we believe you, the nurse, can develop most fully your levels of Rhetorical Sensitivity.

. . . At Least One of Whom Has a Distinct Purpose in Reference to the Other

In the context of our definition, all two-party interactions are not interviews. To be an interview, a two-party interaction must contain at least one party who has a preconceived, specific purpose that somehow affects or seeks from the other. An example of a two-party interaction that would not be an interview is the following: A nurse and a maternity patient's husband, both attempting simply to "pass the time," engage in social conversation about their individual experiences on Okinawa during the Viet Nam War. This situation would not be an interview, according to our definition, because neither party would have a distinct purpose in reference to the other that they were attempting to achieve.

However, most nursing two-party interactions *are* interviews. The nurse may be seeking information from a patient, about a patient, about nursing procedures or medication orders, or the nurse may be attempting to get a patient or other health care professional to do something. Likewise, others may be seeking information from a nurse or attempting to have the nurse perform some procedure, take some action, etc. In other words, in most nursing two-party interaction at least one party has a distinct purpose in reference to the other.

. . . and Both of Whom Speak and Listen from Time to Time

In an interview, both parties speak and listen. The stimuli which one party transmit (the act of speaking) and the stimuli which the other party receive (the act of listening) can be in the form of spoken words and/or nonverbal cues. Communication (and interviewing) does not just involve spoken words but it also involves nonverbal aspects. Later in this chapter we will discuss nonverbal communication in some detail, but for now it is simply important for you to realize that you can be involved in an interview even if spoken words are not used by either or both parties.

FIGURE 2 Nursing Interview Log

	Other Party	Purpose of Interview	Outcome of Interview
1.			
2.			
3.			
4.			
5.			
6.			
7.			
8.			
9.			
10.			

YOUR INVOLVEMENT IN NURSING INTERVIEWS

With our definition of interviewing in mind, take a single sheet of paper and use the format of Figure 2 (page 28) to list some of the interviews in which you were involved the last time you performed your nursing duties. List the other party, and briefly list the purpose of the interview and the outcome of the interview in the spaces provided.

Most of you probably discovered that the space available on your paper allowed you to list only a small percentage of your daily nursing interviews. In a normal working day, it is not uncommon for a nurse to be involved in scores of interviews.

In nursing interviews, one party is the interviewer and one party is the interviewee. The interviewer is generally regarded as the person who initiates the interview and controls the interview; the interviewee is the person from whom information is sought or who is to be persuaded. Before we proceed, turn to the Nursing Interview Log you just completed. Mark each situation with an *R* if you believe you were the interviewer in that situation or *E* if you believe you were the interviewee.

Upon completing this exercise, did you find that in situations involving nurse/patient, nurse/nursing subordinate, and nurse/patient family member, you marked yourself as the *R*; in situations involving nurse/physician, nurse/nursing superior, nurse/administrator or director, you marked yourself as the *E*? The tendency is for us to perceive ourselves as the interviewer if we perceive ourselves in the role superior position, and as the interviewee if we perceive ourselves in the role subordinate position.

Classifying ourselves as interviewers or interviewees according to role relationships is a very great hindrance to being effective communicators and is contrary to the notion of Rhetorical Sensitivity. In most nursing situations, regardless of role relationships, you can be the most Rhetorically Sensitive and the most effective communicator if you assume the position of the interviewer. There are situations in which you should be the interviewee; however, most nursing interview situations, as we shall see in this chapter and the next two chapters, dictate that to be an effective nursing communicator, you should be the interviewer. Also, keep in mind that interviewing roles are *not* fixed. Often in interviews we alternate between being the interviewer and interviewee.

What does it mean for you to be an interviewer? It means that *before each interview situation*, you should ask yourself the questions contained in Figure 3. If you do this, you have taken the first step toward becoming more Rhetorically Sensitive.

You may think asking these questions before each interview entails a lot of trouble and requires hard work. And you would be absolutely correct. It is a demanding and difficult exercise but it is necessary if you

---
FIGURE 3 Pre-Interview Nursing Questions

What is the general purpose of this interview?
What are my specific goals in this interview?
What are ways in which I can achieve these goals?
Out of all the ways I could achieve my goals, what is the best way for the other person *and* for myself to achieve these goals?
---

hope to be an effective communicator. Let's examine these fundamental pre-interview questions.

What is the general purpose of this interview? The general purpose of most nursing interviews can be classified as informative, persuasive, or supportive. In informative interviews, a need or problem is identified and facts are obtained or given or procedures are explained or clarified. In persuasive interviews, a person is shown why something is necessary to be done, how to do it, and is convinced that he or she should do it. In supportive interviews, a person is encouraged to express her or his feelings and concerns to someone who is able to understand and appreciate those feelings and concerns. Later in this book, you will have the opportunity to experience these general purposes in actual nursing situations.

What are my specific goals in this interview? The specific goals of each interview are unique to that interview. No two interviews ever have exactly the same specific goals. Also, most nursing interviews have more than one specific goal. For example, in the same interview you may have as your first specific goal getting a reluctant patient to take prescribed medication and a second specific goal of building trust between you and the patient.

What are the ways in which I can achieve these goals? In most situations there are many different ways to achieve the goal. In an example of a patient reluctant to take medication, what could you do if the medication was vital for the patient's well-being? While the patient has the right to refuse medication, should you simply report the problem to a physician, should you attempt to explain why the medication is necessary, or should you attempt to coerce or force the patient to take the medication? There are many potential ways that the goal of having the patient take the medication could be accomplished.

Out of all the ways I could achieve my goals, what is the best way for the other person and for myself to achieve these goals? While there are usually many ways to achieve any goal, these different ways have different effects and different consequences. What we are advocating, and will stress throughout the book, is that, in nursing interview situations, it is the interviewer's (that is, usually your) responsibility to search through all of the communicative alternatives to achieve specific nursing goals, and select the best alternative that will meet the nursing demands, the needs of the other person, *and* maintain your own self-integrity.

In the example of the patient reluctant to take the medication, what is the best way to achieve your goal? Before answering this question, we must consider some of the issues already discussed. What is the general purpose of the interview? Is it informative, persuasive, or supportive? The answer to this question is: "It depends." It depends on your individual values, beliefs, and judgments. In almost all nursing interviews, you must make a professional judgment of what is the general purpose of the interview.

Most of you would probably make the judgment that the general purpose in our example is to persuade—persuade the patient to take the medication. However, circumstances might be such that the most appropriate general purpose might be to be supportive—if you are supportive, the patient would voluntarily take the medication. Or the most appropriate general purpose might be to be informative—if you inform the patient of reasons for the medication, the patient would willingly take the medication. Perhaps the most appropriate general purpose might be a combination of our types such as informative and supportive.

Once the general purpose has been determined, then the specific purposes should be considered. In the above example, one specific purpose is to have the patient take the medication. Are there any other specific purposes? There may be one or more other specific purposes such as the one mentioned earlier—building trust between you and the patient.

Once the general purpose and specific purpose have been determined, we must search through the alternatives to attaining these purposes and select the best alternative for the particular situation. In our medication example, what is the best alternative? Again, all we can say is: "It depends."

It also must be pointed out at this point that once general purpose, specific purpose, and alternative solutions have been determined prior to the interview, they may, and often do, change during the course of the interview. What if the patient was allergic to the medication but you were initially unaware of this condition? What if there had been a medication error and the medicine was really for another patient with the same last name (or same name)? You can probably see that there are no simple answers to interviewing problems.

With all of this uncertainty, all of these "it depends," is there anything that can be stated definitively about nursing interviews? Yes, one concrete suggestion can be made. A universal statement about all nursing interviews is the following: In order for you to be successful in nursing interviews you must exhibit CONSTANT ADAPTIVE BEHAVIOR—the heart of Rhetorical Sensitivity. You must continually be assessing communicative choices and making professional judgments about the consequences of enacting such choices.

INTERVIEWING STRATEGIES AVAILABLE TO NURSES

To help you implement decisions made during the pre-interview analysis, there are three primary general interviewing strategies that you can employ. A particular strategy may be very appropriate in one situation and very inappropriate in another situation. The three strategies are: directive, nondirective, and combination approaches.

Directive Strategy

A directive strategy is one in which you tell the interviewee what the problem is, what to do, and/or what is expected. You know what you hope to accomplish and how to accomplish it. You are in complete control of the interview. Directive strategies are often appropriate for giving or receiving nursing orders, taking patient histories, explaining nursing procedures, describing patient problems, and, in some cases, counseling situations.

Because the interviewer asks only needed questions, directive strategies are efficient means for obtaining information. However, directive strategies have severe limitations and problems. One of the primary limitations is that such strategies, to be effective, require the interviewer to be an expert—the interviewer must be knowledgeable and competent concerning the subject matter or problem discussed in the interview. Another limitation is that information obtained during the interview is very restrictive—if the proper questions are not asked, necessary information may not be obtained.

Nondirective Strategy

A nondirective strategy is one in which you do *not* tell the interviewee what the problem is, what to do, and/or what is expected. You still control the overall interview by giving encouragement and support when appropriate but allow the interviewee to talk about what the interviewee desires.

Nondirective strategies can be used by nurses in a wide range of information gathering or nursing service situations.

Psychologist Carl Rogers who is regarded as the "Father of Nondirective Counseling" makes the assumption that the interviewee is capable, if given the chance, of identifying and solving her or his own problem. What is needed for the interviewee to be successful in problem identification and solving is for the interviewer to be empathetic with the interviewee. Empathetic means to respond to the interviewee in such a manner as to convey total understanding. You, as interviewer, attempt to become one with the interviewee and make no comments concerning the accuracy or value of statements made by the interviewee. You simply encourage the interviewee to express her or his feelings and attempt to understand those feelings.

While nondirective strategies are very valuable for obtaining the true feelings of interviewees, they also have some limitations and problems. One of the primary limitations is that you do not know what type of information will be obtained. Also, there is no absolute guarantee that the interviewee is, in fact, capable of providing the needed information or solutions. Nondirective interviews are very time-consuming and emotionally demanding on you as interviewer. Since the interviewee is allowed to talk about anything, much extraneous information may be obtained.

Combination Strategy

A combination strategy is one that mixes directive and nondirective strategies and is probably the most useful approach for most nursing situations.

Seldom can you afford the time and demands of nondirective interviews. However, there may be situations such as those involving a client's psychological problems when you, to be successful, will have to employ a "pure" nondirective approach.

Likewise because nursing involves both physical and psychological aspects, a directive strategy will many times not result in optimal outcomes especially when dealing with patients/clients. The fears, beliefs, and values of patients must be considered—something that is difficult to attain using a directive strategy. However, some situations such as routine fact finding, information giving, or emergency situations might dictate a very directive interview. For example, a parent calls and states a child has eaten the contents of a medicine bottle. You must employ a very directive strategy to determine the type of medicine, the amount, and the time at which it was taken.

IMPLEMENTATION OF NURSING INTERVIEW STRATEGIES

Having talked about the general strategies you can employ in interviews, the question is: "How can these strategies be implemented?" These strategies are put into practice through your use of statements and questions.

Statements

There are three basic types of statements you can potentially make in any interview. These statements have been labeled and defined by general semanticist S. I. Hayakawa (1964) as follows: *Reports* are facts capable of verification. *Inferences* are statements about the unknown made on the basis of the known. *Judgments* are expressions of people's approval or disapproval of the occurrences, persons, or objects being described.

In the following examples, identify the example as being a report, inference, or judgment; rate as high, medium, or low the potential for accurate nursing assessment and/or intervention by you if another health care provider had made the statement to you. Finally, briefly state what your next action would be.

EXAMPLE 1: During the past two hours, the maternity patient's blood pressure has increased from 130/80 to 150/100. During that time she has dilated from 5 cm. to 7 cm. Deep Tendon Reflexes are 4+.
Type of Statement: _____
Potential for Accurate Nursing Assessment/Intervention:
   HIGH _____ , MEDIUM _____ , LOW _____
Your Next Action: _____

EXAMPLE 2: Every time the patient's brother has visited, the patient has become depressed afterward. His brother is visiting now, so he'll probably be depressed the rest of the day.
Type of Statement: _____
Potential for Accurate Nursing Assessment/Intervention:
   HIGH _____ , MEDIUM _____ , LOW _____
Your Next Action: _____

EXAMPLE 3: Because the patient is a three-year-old, we'll have to put him in a "papoose bag" before the cut on his chin can be stitched. If he were four, we might be able to reason with him so the bag wouldn't be necessary. But you can't reason with a three-year-old.
Type of Statement: _____
Potential for Accurate Nursing Assessment/Intervention:
   HIGH _____ , MEDIUM _____ , LOW _____
Your Next Action: _____

Example 1 is a report: it contains facts capable of verification. If the report was verified, the potential for accurate assessment/intervention would be high. To a maternity nurse, the report should indicate preeclampsia and the need for a physician's order to administer magnesium sulfate. Continued close observation by a nurse would be required.

Example 2 is an inference; the person making the statement projected what would happen in the future based on what has happened in the past. The potential for accurate assessment/intervention is, at best, medium because you do not know exactly what will happen. The inference is logical to make, however, it must not be treated as fact. If you treat the inference as a report, but the inference is not correct, serious problems could result. For example, if the patient is not depressed after his brother's visit, but you assume he is depressed and treat him as such, the patient may indeed become depressed—not because of his brother but rather because of you. The proper communicative action in this particular case would be to simply observe and make no intervention/assessment unless future behaviors of the patient indicated a need for intervention.

Example 3 is a judgment; a child has been stereotyped and judged to be "unreasonable" and further thought has been stopped by the health care provider. Accurate assessment/intervention is unknown, with a potential for it to be very low. If you acted in accord with the statement (as did a nurse in an actual example observed by your author), the severe restraints of a "papoose bag" would be forced on the child, whereas if the child had been four, such restraints may not have been used. In the actual example, based on the reactions of the child, the forcing on of the "papoose bag" was much more traumatic for the child than was the suturing procedure. If you refrain from making the judgment, much trauma for the child possibly could be avoided. The proper communicative action in this case would be for you to attempt to explain the procedure to the child and observe his reaction—you may find that, given the chance, the child may be more cooperative than many adults.

We are not saying that there are no circumstances where the "papoose bag" in our example would be appropriate. For example, the nature of the laceration may have been such that total immobilization was a medical necessity. What we are saying is that judgments must be made cautiously, and a judgment based on something like one year difference in age is very inappropriate.

If you are using a directive interviewing strategy, you should make statements that are reports. Inferences should be avoided as much as possible, but if used, must be clearly identified as inferences. You should avoid making judgments but there are times when *professional* judgments are necessary based on medical facts.

In nondirective interviewing strategies, you should refrain from making personal reports, inferences, or judgments and should attempt to help the interviewee identify the types of statements she or he is making. Inferences made by the interviewee can be the cause of conflict; judgments made by the interviewee stop the interviewee's thought process; it is only on reports that the interviewee can act to improve her or his situation.

Questions

There have been a number of ways devised to label and classify questions. The basic scheme we will use is based, in part, on a classification made by Gary Richetto and Joseph Zima (1976).

Open Questions. Open questions are very broad and basically unstructured. They indicate the topic to be discussed and allow the interviewee to respond as she or he pleases. Open questions are good for you to use at the beginning of interviews, especially interviews in which nondirective strategies are employed. Open questions are also effective during the course of interviews whenever new topics are brought up, or when the information sought is likely to be threatening or embarrassing. Such questions will allow interviewees to reveal what they feel comfortable revealing at that particular time and they also serve to strengthen the tie between you and the interviewee by allowing you to express rapport or agreement. In addition, open questions help you learn about basic beliefs, values, and attitudes of the interviewee.

> Examples: "Could you tell me about yourself?"
> "Do you have any problems or complaints about the ward?"

Direct Questions. Direct questions ask for explanations about or further expansion of a particular point. Direct questions are appropriate when you need specific replies to specific topics. Such questions limit the freedom of the interviewee response because they specify the desired topic areas. While direct questions are used in nondirective and directive strategies, the more nondirective the interview, the fewer the number of direct questions generally used.

> Examples: "What treatment have you received for this condition?"
> "Could you describe the pain you have been having?"

Closed Questions. Closed questions are a restricted form of direct questions in that they place limits on the range of possible answers the interviewee can give. Often the interviewee is given a list of possible answers to choose from. Such questions allow classification of information and also allow the interviewee to express strengths of opinions or attitudes. Closed questions are seldom used in nondirective strategies but are often a major questioning technique in directive interviews.

> Examples: "Which of the following is the most important nursing role?
> (A) emotional support of patients,
> (B) being a cooperative member of the total health-care team,
> (C) documentation of patient care,
> (D) physical assessment of patients,
> (E) doing routine but necessary chores to provide safety and comfort for patients."
> "Do you think this change in the work schedule will help, hinder, or have no effect on morale?"

Yes/No Questions. Yes/No questions are the most extreme form of direct questions narrowing the range of possible answers to one of two choices. A question is classified as a yes/no question anytime the response can be yes or no, or anytime a respondent is asked to choose between two alternatives. Such questions are useful in obtaining needed factual data. Like closed questions, yes/no questions are used often in directive interviews but seldom in nondirective interviews.

> Examples: "Have you had any previous heart trouble?"
> "Kathy, you've been working here a year. We're interested in knowing whether you're satisfied or dissatisfied with your present job."

Probes. Probes are questions used to followup other questions or statements, or to get further information on particular points. Such questions allow the interviewee to enlarge, clarify, or explain a particular response made, and allow you to focus discussion on specific content and avoid unnecessary information. Probes are perhaps the most useful type of questions for you in any type of interviewing strategy. While there are many forms of probes, all probes provide you the opportunity to attempt to get specific, complete responses from your interviewee.

> Examples: "What do you mean?"
> "Could you tell me more about how you felt yesterday?"

Restatements. Restatements act as an echo or mirror for the interviewee. When you repeat exactly what was said by the interviewee or paraphrase what was said, you allow the interviewee to hear her or his own words which is often very revealing for the interviewee. This technique also demonstrates interviewer empathy for the interviewee, and is a check on listening accuracy and perception accuracy for both you and the interviewee. After a restatement by you, the interviewee has the opportunity to respond: "Yes, that's what I meant," or "No, what I meant was . . ." Restatements are a very valuable tool for you in nondirective interviewing strategies.

> Examples: "What you've said is you're unhappy with the care you've received."
> "If I understand you correctly, you're saying that the pain medication doesn't seem to be helping you."

In conjunction with restatements, two additional responses need to be mentioned as types of questions important for you as a nurse, especially whenever a nondirective strategy is employed. These questions may not initially be considered by you to be questions but we prefer to call them questions because they often seek and/or elicit response from the interviewee.

Mm-hm. The sound "mm-hm" or a similar sound, although not a word, is a verbal response. Such sounds can be used by you in nondirective strategies for many purposes. "Mm-hm," like restatements, can tell the interviewee that you understand and are empathetic. It can also indicate your approval of what is being said by the interviewee, and it can indicate to the interviewee that she or he should continue talking. In addition, such a sound may imply criticism or it may suggest that you want to hear more before commenting or questioning further. While a very valuable technique, the use of "mm-hm" is often abused by nurses in interviews with patients/clients. You should keep in mind that "mm-hm" may be perceived by the interviewee in multiple manners. "Mm-hm" should be used, but used discreetly, and only when necessary.

Silence. Another valuable technique, but one that many nurses do not use enough, is silence. Silence is often the most important thing you can do to attain success in nondirective interviews, especially ones involving a counseling situation. Recall that an assumption of nondirective strategies is that, given the chance, the interviewee can identify and solve her or his own problems. A natural human tendency in an interview is to dislike silence. When there is silence, a person has a desire to say something, anything, to break the silence. Very often, an interviewee who has a problem or concern will break silence by talking about what is most important to that person at that particular time—the problem or concern. Silence may be uncomfortable but it can be used by you to get responses that otherwise could not be obtained.

Leading Questions. One additional type question should be discussed. This type question, a leading question, is a question that implies a correct response in the question.

Example: "That is how you feel, isn't it?"

Often it is stated that leading questions should always be avoided. Our position is that in nursing communication, leading questions should generally be avoided, however, there are situations when they are necessary. When the patient's welfare is at stake, leading questions by you may be very appropriate. For example, a rehabilitation nurse has a patient who needs movement or else risks complications such as formation of blood clots. In such a case, a very appropriate leading question by the nurse could be: "You will get up and walk with me, won't you?"

A summary of the basic questions, their primary purposes (what they can accomplish), and what type of strategies can best incorporate them is contained in Figure 4.

So far in this chapter we have discussed the importance of interviewing for you, the nurse, the general strategies available for nursing interviews, and the general types of questions you can ask in an interview. Now we'll examine how the types of questions can be incorporated into the general strategies.

FIGURE 4 Summary of Basic Interviewing Questions

Type question	Primary purposes	Primary strategies used in
open	begin interview, introduce new topics, get threatening or embarrassing information, build rapport, learn about basic beliefs, values, attitudes	nondirective, combination
direct	get specific replies to specific topics	directive, combination
closed	limit range of possible answers, classify information, express strengths of opinions or attitudes	directive, combination
yes/no	allow one of two choices, obtain factual data	directive
probes	followup other questions, get further information on particular points, enlarge, clarify or explain, focus discussion on specific content	directive, nondirective, combination
restatements	act as echo or mirror, show empathy, check listening and perceptions	nondirective, combination
"mm-hm"	show understanding and/or empathy, may indicate approval and/or criticism, may signal the interviewee to continue	nondirective, combination
silence	allow interviewee to speak, allow interviewee to express intimate or deep feelings	nondirective, combination
leading	generally to be avoided, use for medical necessities	directive

Interviewing Schedules

Prior to planning the exact wording of questions, you must consider the general purpose, specific purpose, and likelihood of success of various alternatives. Having determined these factors, you must then determine what strategy would fulfill your purpose. You can implement the strategy you choose using one of four plans called *interviewing schedules*—a schedule being the manner in which questions will be asked. The four schedules are labeled: nonscheduled, moderately scheduled, highly scheduled, and highly scheduled standardized.

Nonscheduled Interviews. A nonscheduled interview is nothing more than an awareness of topics and subtopics that potentially could be discussed. Exact type or wording of questions is not planned although the overall strategy is planned. Although nonscheduled interviews are the types of interviews most likely conducted by nurses in all types of nursing situations, they should not be as widely used as they are. Whenever possible, to be an effective communicator, you should attempt to select a schedule with more structure than a nonscheduled interview.

Moderately Scheduled Interviews. In a moderately scheduled interview the major questions to be asked and possible probing questions are considered *before* the interview occurs. It is the type of schedule we would recommend for most nursing interviews. A moderately scheduled interview allows you a great deal of freedom in the interview but it also imposes a structure on the interview which is likely to increase your credibility in the eyes both of the interviewee *and* yourself, and which will help ensure that the objectives of the interview are attained.

The interviews conducted with nurses that are used in this book are moderately scheduled interviews. The major questions and possible probes were prepared before the interviews began and are presented in Figure 5. During the course of the interview, additional probes and modifications were made depending upon the information obtained during the interview.

Highly Scheduled Interviews. In a highly scheduled interview the precise wording of all the questions to be asked is determined prior to the interview and usually the questions are written out in exactly the manner in which they will be asked. Such an interview allows no flexibility by you and is applicable only when a directive strategy is employed. Highly scheduled interviews are often used in taking patient histories.

FIGURE 5 Nursing Interview Questionnaire

Questions for interviews of nurses

Nursing degree(s), Years experience as nurse, Area of nursing, Job title, Organization

What is your perception of the role of the nurse? Has that perception changed since you started working? How? How do you see the status of nurses? Has this perception changed since you started working? How?

What are the primary communication demands on nurses? What is effective nursing communication?

What formal training do you have in communication? What communication skills are most necessary for you in your job? In what communication skills do you wish you had more training?

With what kinds of patients do you most often interact? What are the most difficult communication problems you have with these types of patients? Could you give an example or two? (Be specific—use of actual examples is best.) Do you have any communication techniques that are most effective for you?

When communicating with nursing peers and subordinates, what types of communication problems do you encounter? Be specific and give actual examples if possible. When communicating with physicians, what types of communication problems do you encounter? Be specific and give actual examples if possible. When communicating with other health care team members such as educators, therapists, technicians, administrators, directors, planners, etc., what types of communication problems do you encounter? (You don't have to answer for all these types, a couple examples will be sufficient.)

Describe instances when you have to communicate as a member of a small group (3 to 12 people)? What types of communication problems do you encounter in such groups? Be specific; use actual examples.

In large health care organizations, what are the main communication problems that you have? Why do you think these problems exist? Are there any communication techniques that seem to work well, from your experience, in large health care organizations? Explain.

Have you ever had to give a public speech involving nursing? To whom? What were your perceptions of the experience?

Highly Scheduled Standardized Interviews. In a highly scheduled standardized interview the exact wording of questions is predetermined and interviewee answer options are also predetermined and included with the questions. Almost all questions in highly scheduled standardized interviews are closed or yes/no questions. Such interviews have limited value to you as a nurse but can be used in situations like surveys in which quantifiable data are needed.

Having considered the schedule of questions to be used in the interview, you must next consider the manner in which questions will be asked, that is, the sequence to be followed.

Interview Sequencing

There are many ways of sequencing questions in an interview. For example, questions can be sequenced in chronological order by topic, or according to a problem-solution format. Another way of sequencing questions is by the types of questions asked. Some commonly used examples of this are as follows: (1) The funnel sequence—in which you start with open questions and progress to more and more direct questions and even ultimately to very closed or yes/no questions; (2) the inverted funnel sequence—in which you begin with very closed questions and progress to more open questions; (3) the tunnel sequence—in which a string of all of the same type of questions are asked, for example, a series of open questions or a series of closed questions. The important point to remember is that some logical order should be attempted to be used in any type of question sequence.

Keeping in mind that some sort of sequencing is desirable in nursing interviews, you should also be aware that the language used in phrasing your questions must be accurate, clear, understandable to the interviewee, and appropriate for the situation. Later, we shall see nursing interview examples in which proper language usage is crucial to achieve satisfactory outcomes.

NONVERBAL COMMUNICATION

Before discussing conduct of specific nursing interviews, we must consider one other important factor. Earlier in this book, we stated that in any interview only one-third of the social meaning is derived from the words that are used, two-thirds of the meaning is derived from nonverbal communication. Just what is nonverbal communication? And what considerations should be made concerning nonverbal communication before and during an interview?

Nonverbal communication is an area of study that has received wide attention in recent years. Many paperback books have been written that claim to give us the secrets of "reading other people like a book," "getting people to do whatever we want them to do," etc. Unfortunately, nonverbal communication is not as simple as many people would like us to believe. Nonverbal communication is very complex.

We will define nonverbal communication simply as all communication in person-to-person interaction except the words themselves.

Many of you may associate the term *nonverbal communication* with body movements. Body movements are but one form of nonverbal communication. In the following pages, several other nonverbal aspects will be discussed. Before stating specifics about the range of nonverbal influences, we will introduce you to this range by discussing several functions that nonverbal communication can serve in reference to the actual words you use in interviews.

Functions of Nonverbal Communication

Nonverbal communication expert Mark L. Knapp (1978) has identified six basic functions nonverbal communication can serve with respect to verbal communication.

Repeating. Nonverbal communication can repeat what you say verbally. For example, if you told a patient to wait in the waiting area and pointed in that direction, you would be repeating nonverbally what you said verbally.

Contradicting. Nonverbal communication can also contradict your verbal behavior. An example of contradicting would be a nurse telling a patient that stopping smoking and weight reduction were critical for the patient's well-being, but the nurse was herself or himself a smoker and obese.

Substituting. Nonverbal behavior can also substitute for your verbal messages. For example, you walk to the nursing station at a very slow pace with shoulders slumped and head low, you don't have to actually say to others, "This has been a rotten day"—the message is conveyed without words.

Complementing. Nonverbal behavior can also modify, or elaborate on, your verbal messages. For example, the nurse who is late for work may reflect an attitude of embarrassment when talking to her or his superior about the reasons for being late.

Accenting. Nonverbal behavior may accent parts of your verbal messages much as underlining words, or italicizing them, serves to emphasize them. Movements of the hands or head are frequently used to accent verbal messages. For example, patients who are angry may often clench their teeth between words and may hit their fists on tables or similar objects.

Regulating. Nonverbal communication is also used to regulate the communication flow between people. When you are talking, you signal others by your head nods, arm movements, and/or shifts in body position that they should continue to speak, or to stop speaking because you want to talk.

These are the six functions that nonverbal communication can serve in reference to the words you actually use. Not only do nonverbal aspects serve functions with respect to verbal but, in accord with our definition, nonverbal aspects are communication by themselves. What concrete suggestions can be made to you, a nurse, concerning use of nonverbal communication?

Using Nonverbal Communication to Attain Nursing Goals

Unlike much of the popular literature, we will *not* make lists of "always do this, never do this" or "this particular nonverbal act always means . . ." Attaching universal meaning to nonverbal communication, while making for interesting reading and perhaps giving you a sense of security, will *not* contribute to more effective nursing communication. In fact, such definitive beliefs about nonverbal meaning will likely make you a less effective communicator and hinder effective patient/client care.

The important thing for you as a nurse to develop is a sensitivity to nonverbal cues. While it is impossible to accurately interpret any single nonverbal cue, by considering clusters of nonverbal cues you can often gain insight into and can control a communicative interaction. It must be pointed out that control is not the same as manipulation—control means being aware of one's self and the existing environment and then using this awareness to more effectively meet the needs of the other person and oneself.

What are the specific elements of nonverbal communication? Figure 6 illustrates a useful way of classifying nonverbal communication devised by Mark Knapp. We will look at these seven dimensions and discuss some issues that you should be aware of as a nurse.

Dimensions of Nonverbal Communication Related to Nursing

Body Motion. When people are communicating, their bodies often convey emotional states. For example, if a patient has excessive movement of the extremities (hands, arms, feet, legs), is reluctant to maintain eye contact (that is, will not look at you in a "normal" manner), and maintains a slouched body position, what does this mean? It means the patient is extremely nervous, doesn't it? It depends! While all the described nonverbal signs may mean nervousness, they may also mean things such as emotional problems, physical pain, or a host of other possibilities.

DISCUSSION QUESTION

What should you do if you note unusual nonverbal body cues from a patient/client?

FIGURE 6 A Classification of Nonverbal Communication

(1) Body Motion
Body motion typically includes gestures, movements of the body, limbs, hands, head, feet and legs, facial expressions, eye behavior, and posture.

(2) Physical Characteristics
Whereas body motion is concerned with movement and motion, physical characteristics include things which remain relatively unchanged such as: physique or body shape, general attractiveness, body or breath odors, height, weight, hair, and skin color or tone.

(3) Touching Behavior
Touching behavior is any type of act in which one person physically touches another person. This can include simple things like handshakes, caresses, or simply "bumping into someone."

(4) Paralanguage
Paralanguage concerns how we say words, not what we say. Things such as pitch, voice rate, intensity, and vocal sounds such as *uh huh, mmm, ahh,* are all included in the category of paralanguage.

(5) Personal Space
Personal space or as it is often called, proxemics, deals with the notion that we are influenced by the spatial relationships between ourselves and other people and also things in our environment.

(6) Artifacts
Artifacts are defined as those objects that are in contact with a person and can be a source of nonverbal stimuli for that person or for someone else. Examples of artifacts are clothes, eyeglasses, wigs and other hairpieces, perfumes, lipstick, and various other adornments of the body.

(7) Environmental Factors
Previous categories all are concerned with appearance and behaviors of persons involved in communicating. However, the environment in which these people communicate also influences communication. Examples of environmental factors are architectural style, furniture, interior decorating, lighting conditions, temperature, smells, colors, and additional noises or music.

You should be sensitive to such nonverbal cues and through *interviewing techniques,* attempt to explore the reasons for the behavior. It is sufficient to recognize that body motion *may* indicate a problem or concern, *not* that it does indicate a particular "abnormality."

You must also be aware of your own body motion and be sensitive to others' perceptions of that motion. In a communicative interaction, you influence the other person just as the other person influences you.

Physical Characteristics. While body motion is changing from moment to moment, physical characteristics remain relatively unchanged over short periods of time. Our basic body construction is fixed except for the long-term effects of aging. Physical characteristics influence communication—we all have biases, prejudices, and stereotypes that affect how we interact with people based on their height, weight, skin or hair color, etc.

DISCUSSION QUESTION

What are some common biases based on physical characteristics?

What is important for you to know is that physical characteristics do influence communication and you must constantly remind yourself of this fact. You must ask, "Am I responding in my communication to the person or to my stereotypes concerning the person's physical characteristics?" Effective nursing communication dictates that we respond to individual people and not to their physical characteristics.

Touching Behavior. Touching may be the most important but least used and understood communicative behavior by nurses, especially when dealing with patients who are infants or children.

Touch can communicate warmth, understanding, affection, nurturing and caring—all basic human needs. Unfortunately societal values have evolved that restrict the use of touch—touch has come to be associated with sexual activity.

Research, reported by Marshall Klaus and John Kennell (1982), indicates that small premature infants who are not touched daily during stays in hospital nurseries will not gain weight or develop as fast as infants who are touched. This need for touch, although suppressed by societal norms, continues throughout life.

In discussing touch, it is appropriate to point out an unresolved controversy in nonverbal communication research—how much of nonverbal communication behavior is inborn in us (i.e., nature), how much is learned (i.e., nurture)? There is no clear answer to this question.

DISCUSSION QUESTION

You have just been handed a newborn infant. How would you hold the infant?

Did you find that you held the baby's head in your left arm and supported the baby's body and legs with your right arm and hand? Why?

No matter which way you held the baby, now switch to the opposite arm. Do you notice anything different? Most of you will find that when the baby's head is held in the left arm, you will hold the baby much closer to your body than if the baby's head is held in the right arm.

Some of you may be saying, "I held the baby's head in my left arm because I'm right-handed and by holding the head in the left arm, it allows me to use my right hand to feed it." In a classroom setting with 29 student nurses, your author attempted this little experiment and all 29 held the baby's head in the left arm even though 12 of the 29 reported being left-handed.

In this example, you are communicating with the baby and the baby is communicating with you. For about nine months prior to birth, a constant stimulus for the baby has been sound—the sound of the mother's heartbeat. Normally for at least the first few weeks after birth, the baby will seek the sound of a human heart. If you hold the baby's head in your left arm, the baby will usually nestle close to your body in order to hear your heartbeat; if you hold the baby's head in your right arm the baby cannot hear your heartbeat and consequently will be likely to squirm and kick and you will naturally hold the baby farther from your body. This is nonverbal communication. You might be tempted to say this is learned communication behavior, however, your author has experienced adults and children who claim to have never held a baby but behave in the same manner as people who are in contact with infants almost daily. Is it nature, nurture, or a combination of the two?

What implications does this example have for you as a nurse? What if you observe a mother holding her newborn child with the child's head in her right arm. Often, *but not always,* such nonverbal communicative behavior, if it is accompanied by the mother's lack of eye contact with the baby, is indicative that the mother is very unsure of her feelings toward the baby and may even indicate that the mother does not want the child. Note that we have stated, "Often, *but not always...*" As stated earlier, you cannot draw universal conclusions based on a single nonverbal communicative act. Such an act should be, however, a signal to you that a situation exists that warrants further observation and indicates a need for exploration through professional interviewing techniques.

Paralanguage. You have probably all heard someone say: "It's not what she said, but how she said it . . . ." "How" we say things is paralanguage. For example, you have just come on duty at a hospital and are making morning rounds with a physician. The physician turns to you and says: "I'm pleased about how well the nursing staff informed me concerning the patient's lack of progress during the night." Depending on the tone, rate, and volume of the physician's voice and the inflections used, you could interpret the statement in two very different ways—the physician was either well informed or the physician was not informed.

Like many other aspects of nonverbal communication, paralanguage can convey emotional or psychological states. But also like other nonverbal dimensions, we cannot claim: "This always means . . ."

What is important for you is to be sensitive to your use of paralanguage and the vocal tones and sounds made by others. You must be willing to explore discrepancies between paralanguage and other nonverbal and verbal components of communication. For example, consider the following: A patient says to you, "I, mmm, am really not, ahh, having, you know, much pain, um, today, I guess." The words by themselves indicate the patient is not experiencing pain; however, the vocalized pauses and fillers (mmm, ahh, you know, um, I guess) may be an indication that the patient is in pain. It is your responsibility to explore if there is a discrepancy.

Personal Space. Personal space or *proxemics* as it is sometimes called is another very important nonverbal communication variable to be considered. Anthropologist Edward Hall (1959) has defined the space around a person according to four categories, which for the American culture are listed in Figure 7.

Normally when conversing with someone, most of us prefer to maintain a casual-personal distance (18 inches to 4 feet). Only when the other is someone with whom we are intimate, will we feel comfortable if our distance is less than 18 inches. If we maintain a social-consultative distance during conversation, we infer the conversation is businesslike and impersonal. We operate in public distance when addressing large groups of people or if the conversation is very impersonal.

Most nurses instinctively maintain appropriate distances when interacting with other nurses, physicians, or other health care professionals. However, when interacting with patients/clients, it is often a different case. The nature of nursing is such that very often it is necessary for you to "invade" the intimate distance of a patient, that is to be closer than 18 inches to the patient. What must be realized is that when the intimate space of a patient is entered, the patient is likely to feel threatened and react defensively.

On the other hand, if you attempt to communicate with a patient at distances greater than four feet, for example, you stand at the doorway

FIGURE 7 Classification of Personal Distances

intimate	actual physical contact to 18 inches
casual-personal	18 inches to 4 feet
social-consultative	4 feet to 12 feet
public	12 feet and beyond

or at the foot of the bed, the patient is likely to perceive you as very nonpersonal and not truly interested in the patient as a person. To be the most effective communicator with patients, you should attempt, whenever reasonably possible, to maintain a distance of 18 inches to 4 feet between yourself and the patient. At this distance, the patient is most likely to perceive you as a caring professional individual.

Maintaining personal space around us is a universal tendency in both humans and animals ("nature"); however, the precise distances vary among cultures ("nurture").

The distances reported in Figure 7 are derived from the "average" American culture. Subcultures in America and different cultures in the world have evolved different distances. In a few cultures, the intimate zone is greater than 18 inches, sometimes extending up to 24 inches or more; in many cultures the intimate zone is less than 18 inches and may be as small as 9 or 12 inches. Have you ever talked to someone from a different culture (e.g., an American talking to someone from the Middle Eastern part of the world) and felt that person was being very pushy, aggressive, and rude? Quite possibly this was simply because her or his intimate zone was much less than yours.

Nurses must be aware that personal distances do affect communication, and there are cultural differences that must be considered and adapted to when communicating with people of other cultures.

Artifacts. Perhaps the most important artifacts in nursing communication are uniforms. The nurse's uniform, the physician's long white coat, the intern's short white coat, the patient's hospital gown (with the open back) all profoundly influence communication by signifying role and status relationships.

While such role and status communication restrictions are often beneficial to nursing communication, there are many times when they are a hindrance. For example, in some instances public health or community nurses will find communication with clients more effective if "civilian" clothes, as opposed to nurse's uniforms, are worn. The lack of uniform can, in some cases, signify to the clients that the nurse is one of them and someone who can be trusted. While no definitive guidelines can be given about such issues, we believe it is something that should at least be considered.

Other artifacts that can have important influences on nursing communication include a nurse's jewelry, strong perfumes or other body scents, long painted fingernails (for female nurses), and other heavy cosmetic enhancements. In addition to, and probably largely because of, creating health problems (for example, spreading infections), such "beautifiers" often hinder effective nursing communication because they are interpreted by others to mean the nurse is nonprofessional.

Environmental Factors. Environmental factors are present in every interaction between people, and while often you can have no control over such factors, many times you can. Even if you cannot control environmental factors, recognizing them and their influence can often allow you to be a more effective communicator.

Most hospital rooms by their architectural design and decor contribute to nonpersonal communication. The typical sterile white walls, the hospital bed, the businesslike chairs, and the medical equipment, while contributing to efficient mechanical medical care, do little to contribute to effective personal communication. By recognizing this influence, you may find that in situations that dictate a high level of personal communication, for example with patients with psychological problems, more effective communication can occur in more conducive environments such as outside in a garden area or in a personal office.

In many situations you have direct control over environmental factors such as furniture placement. Consider the following example.

DISCUSSION QUESTION

You, the nurse, are in an office seated behind a desk which is in the middle of a room. Your job involves communicating with clients. Where would you place the client's chair? Does it make any difference where the chair is placed?

It makes a great deal of difference where the chair is placed. If the chair is placed on the opposite side of the desk, a strict role superior/subordinate relationship is implied which is likely to result in very impersonal, businesslike communicative interaction. If the chair is placed to the side of the desk, a less formal setting is created which is likely to result in more personal communication but still with a degree of formality. If the chair is placed such that the desk does not come between you and the client, an informal atmosphere is implied which can result in very personal, informal communication. Which situation is best? Once again it depends on the situation and the purposes of the interview.

An entire book could be devoted to nonverbal communication in nursing. What has been attempted here is just a brief overview. It is hoped that this overview will make you a little more aware of the extent and importance of nonverbal communication in nursing situations.

SUMMARY

In this chapter, interviews are identified as often the most important communicative configuration facing you as a nurse. We defined an interview as: two people, at least one of whom has a distinct purpose in reference to the other, and both of whom speak and listen from time to time.

While detailing the implications of this interviewing definition, we highlighted the range of nursing interviews. Pre-interview considerations necessary for you to enact Rhetorical Sensitivity principles were discussed. Focus was placed on constant adaptive behavior in your nursing interviews.

Strategies you can use during nursing interviews were identified as directive, nondirective, and combination approaches. Statements labeled reports, inferences, and judgments were defined and their effects on nursing interviews discussed. The terms open, direct, closed, yes/no, probe, restatement, mm-hm, silence, and leading were applied to questions, and use of these questions was explored in the context of nursing interviews. Importance of scheduling and sequencing in your interviews was stressed.

A presentation was made concerning the role of nonverbal communication in nursing interviews. Nonverbal communication was defined as all communication in person-to-person interaction except the words themselves. Functions that nonverbal communication can serve, in reference to the words you use, were identified as repeating, contradicting, substituting, complementing, accenting, and regulating. Finally, the nonverbal dimensions of body motion, physical characteristics, touching behavior, paralanguage, personal space, artifacts, and environmental factors were related to nursing interviews.

This chapter has provided considerations, tools, and techniques that you can use to implement the construct of Rhetorical Sensitivity discussed in Chapter 1. In Chapter 3 we shall attempt to have you put into practice the constructs and concepts discussed so far in the context of nurse-patient/client interviews.

References

Goyer, R. S., Redding, W. C., & Rickey, J. T. *Interviewing principles and techniques: A project text.* Dubuque, Iowa: Wm. C. Brown Publishers, 1968, p. 6.

Hall, E. T. *The silent language.* New York: Doubleday & Co., 1959.

Hayakawa, S. I. *Language in thought and action* (2nd ed.). New York: Harcourt, Brace & World, Inc., 1964, pp. 38-44.

Klaus, M. H., & Kennell, J. H. *Parent-infant bonding* (2nd ed.). St. Louis: The C. V. Mosby Company, 1982, p. 164.

Knapp, M. L. *Nonverbal communication in human interaction* (2nd ed.). New York: Holt, Rinehart and Winston, 1978, pp. 12-26.

Richetto, G. M., & Zima, J. P. *Fundamentals of interviewing.* Modules in Speech Communication. Palo Alto, California: Science Research Associates, Inc., 1976.

Rogers, C. R. *Client-centered therapy.* Boston: Houghton Mifflin Company, 1965.

Suggested Readings

Interviewing

Richetto, G. M., & Zima, J. P. *Fundamentals of interviewing* (2nd ed.). Modules in Speech Communication. Palo Alto, California: Science Research Associates, Inc., 1981.
A condensed overview of the interviewing process. Identifies major interviewing variables including strategies, questions, and probing techniques. Also discusses common problems encountered in interviews.

Stewart, C. J., & Cash, W. B. *Interviewing principles and practices* (3rd ed.). Dubuque, Iowa: Wm. C. Brown Company Publishers, 1982.
Application of communication theory to the interviewing process. Specifics on a wide range of interview types such as informational, persuasive, employment, performance appraisal, and counseling.

Nonverbal Communication

Knapp, M. L. *Nonverbal communication in human interaction* (2nd ed.). New York: Holt, Rinehart and Winston, 1978.
The most comprehensive treatment of nonverbal communication available. Soundly based on research findings and well documented. Easy and enjoyable reading.

Knapp, M. L. *Essentials of nonverbal communication.* New York: Holt, Rinehart and Winston, 1980.
A condensed version of Knapp's *Nonverbal communication in human interaction.* Highlights major dimensions and research findings in nonverbal communication.

CHAPTER 3

Communicating with Patients

If you understand your communicative attitudes, learn interviewing skills, and understand verbal and nonverbal influences, will you be an effective communicator? Not necessarily. Our definition of communication involves other crucial considerations. Those considerations are Other and interaction with Other.

For you as a nurse, the most important Other is a patient or client. If there were no clients, there would be no nurses; if there was no communication between clients and nurses, technical and mechanical nursing skills and procedures would often be inefficient, ineffective, and/or inaccurate. Successful nursing is often successful communication between nurse and patient/client.

COMMUNICATIVE NEEDS OF PATIENTS/CLIENTS

You are not the same as any other nurse—your individual attitudes, beliefs, values, experiences, and abilities are unique. In addition, you are different from day to day, moment to moment.

Likewise, each patient/client and each situation is unique and constantly changing. Communicative techniques successful with one patient may not be successful with another patient or even with the same patient at a different time or by a different nurse.

There may be situations in which nursing communicative techniques you learned as "good" may be "bad," and other times when "bad" techniques may be "good." Consider the following example described by Ruth Searight (1980): "We nurses always thought being professional meant never venting our anger or frustration in front of a patient. But then we met Gary Maine, a quadriplegic with chronic schizophrenia. To help Gary get in touch with *his* feelings, we had to let *our* feelings show."

Searight goes on to explain how she and other nurses employed empathic and therapeutic technique after technique in an attempt to help Gary—all attempts meeting with failure. Gary would not cooperate; he would do everything he could to rebel and disrupt the nursing plan.

Finally, Searight states: "I did what I thought I'd never do—I lost my temper. 'Gary, if you don't drink this juice, you'll be wearing it.' I'll admit my approach was unprofessional. But Gary looked at me as if seeing me for the first time, and he actually *laughed*—for the first time. Then he drank the juice." Further nursing interactions with Gary showed that, in many instances, only by the nurses expressing their "real feelings" could they get Gary to cooperate.

This example is but one of many in which "poor" nursing practice is actually the best nursing practice.

If we consider the uniqueness of each nurse, each patient/client, each situation, how can we present any guidelines for you to follow? In a sense, we cannot. Only you can provide your own guidelines. Further, these guidelines can only be developed through experience and hard work in each of your nursing encounters.

To help you develop experience and communicative habits of hard work, later in this chapter we shall present an exercise that we have employed several times in workshops and in-services for nursing students and practicing nurses. Before we put you to work, we want to briefly present a few concepts concerning interaction with an Other in an interview and responsibilities you have to that Other during the course of an interview. Your understanding of these concepts is important if you desire to implement Rhetorical Sensitivity.

The Social Penetration Process

Irwin Altman and Dalmas Taylor (1973) have described the manner in which we get to know other people. A conceptualization of their scheme is diagrammed in Figure 8.

FIGURE 8 The Social Penetration Process

A Person's Personality, Attitudes, Beliefs, Opinions, etc.

Learned upon initial contact

Learned as we get to "know" a person

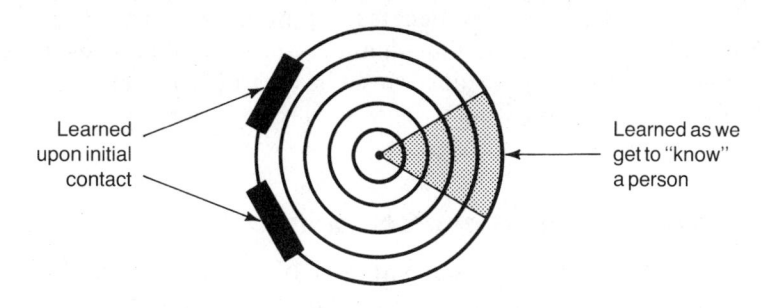

Imagine that each person's personality structure is like an onion. An onion is composed of various layers. Upon initial inspection, all you see is the onion's outer layer. As you peel off the outer layers, the inner layers are revealed and the onion's odor becomes stronger. Analogously, when you first meet a client, all that can be determined is the peripheral aspects of the client's personality. As you and the client communicate, more central aspects of the client's personality are revealed.

The process of exploring outer layers before exploring inner layers is a natural human ritual and if this ritual is violated, communication is likely to be ineffective. For example, consider how you would react if a total stranger walked up to you and asked, "How is your sex life?" Reactions of most of us would be unprintable. Now consider if a lifelong intimate friend asked you the same question. For most of us, our reaction would be very different, however, some of us would react in a similar manner as we would to the stranger. Why these reactions?

The stranger is violating the social penetration process by asking a question that concerns an area, that for most, is a very inner personal layer and the stranger knows nothing about our outer layers. Your lifelong friend may have progressed to the point where necessary outer layers have been revealed. However, for some the question of sexual satisfaction is at the very core of personality. Each of us orders our layers in an individual manner—what is central for one person may not be so central for another. Aspects of our core personality can be so personal that, in a lifetime, we will reveal them to few, if any, people. Each of us can think of things about ourselves that we would never tell another person.

Why is the social penetration process so important for nurse-patient communication? Often, medical situations are such that you must obtain information that lies in the inner core for a patient. Medical considerations could be so critical that information is needed at once. However, many nurses acquire that habit of "going right to the core" with all patients. We are advocating that, whenever possible, you must conduct an orderly social penetration process if you hope to be a successful communicator. You should, when circumstances allow, take the time and effort to explore outer layers of a patient's personality before attempting to explore the inner layers.

The Co-Orientation Perspective

Perceptions are an important variable in communication. Perceptions are particularly important in nurse-patient/client communication. You have perceptions of the patient; the patient has perceptions of you. In addition, each has perceptions of the perceptions of the other; that is, each has meta-perceptions (meta meaning beyond). If this isn't complicated enough, each also has meta-meta perceptions (perceptions of the other's perceptions of the self's perceptions), and so forth.

For example, you have a conversation with a female patient one day postoperative after a hysterectomy. You perceive the patient. The patient perceives you perceiving her. You, in turn, perceive her perceiving you perceiving her. You both communicate these various levels of perceptions even though neither often consciously thinks of these factors.

According to a perspective called Co-Orientation, each perception, meta-perception, meta-meta perception, etc., has two primary dimensions—the dimensions of *accuracy* and of *agreement*. Researchers such as R. D. Laing, H. Phillipson, and A. R. Lee (1966) have detailed the effects of various degrees of perceptual accuracy and agreement. It is beyond our scope to extensively discuss this area of psychological research; however, it is important to give some rudimentary consideration.

Consider the example of the postoperative hysterectomy patient. In your conversation with her, you perceive she is concerned about a vaginal discharge she is having. You examine her, and, based on your examination, are concerned the discharge could signal a complication (such as an infection). She is concerned about the discharge, and you are concerned about the discharge. Under these circumstances, both of you would have perceptions high in accuracy and high in agreement. Results from this situation are most likely what we call "communication" and "constructive relationship."

However, if the patient is having the discharge and perceives it as being serious, and you recognize the discharge but perceive it as being normal, the two of you would have high accuracy (there is a discharge) but low agreement (she thinks it is serious; you think it is not serious).

The most likely result of such a state would be what we call "conflict." *Conflict* as we have used the term is not necessarily negative. From conflict, communication and constructive relationships can result.

Next consider the following case: You perceive the patient as being concerned and she, in fact, is concerned (high agreement). However, she is concerned about the discharge; you think she is concerned about some other factor, such as how her husband will react to her because she has lost a body part associated with her sexuality (low accuracy). In this case, the most likely result of such perceptions we call "ignorance" and the potential for your taking inappropriate action is great, as is the potential for destructive relationships between you and the patient.

Finally, consider a case in which, based upon comments the patient has made to you, you perceive her as thinking that her husband will be very accepting and supportive. However, in her comments, the patient was attempting to tell you about her feelings of uncertainty concerning how her husband will react sexually to her. In such a situation, there is low accuracy (you each perceive the meaning of the message differently) and there is low agreement (she is concerned, you are not). Such a state is extremely dangerous for the result is often for both parties to think they are in *high agreement* and *high accuracy*. We call this a "double negative effect" and, if it occurs, the most likely results are a limiting of active thought processes, a limiting of communication, and an increase in potential for serious problems in both terms of actions and relationships between nurse and patient.

In an actual example, a patient was perceived by all the nurses caring for her as accepting her hysterectomy very well—joking, commenting on the "anti-rape whistle" she had been given as a gift. However, when the patient was alone she cried because of her feelings of loss of sexuality and concern about her husband's potential reactions. A nurse friend of the patient, upon visiting, brought a small gift of French chocolates and said, "I really don't know how you're reacting to your operation. I know many women feel very depressed because of the hormonal changes and loss of a sexual body part. I brought you chocolates because I read that chocolates are supposed to give women a mood lift if they're feeling low. Also, I know you like chocolate." The patient looked at the friend, burst into tears, and proceeded to tell the friend how low she was feeling, about her crying episodes, and about her feelings concerning her husband's acceptance. In this actual incident, the staff nurses developed perceptions of low accuracy and low agreement in reference to the patient's perceptions, but the nurse friend was able to form perceptions high in accuracy and high in agreement with the patient's perceptions. The difference in potential for helping the patient should be obvious.

It is important for you to recognize that nursing interviews are most likely to be successful when both parties' perceptions are accurate—

when both parties can understand what the other person is thinking and saying. No matter if they agree or disagree with each other, as long as they have accurate understanding of each other, they can successfully communicate. In nurse/patient interviews it is also important to keep in mind that patients' "consumer awareness" has generally been increasing. As one nurse commented, "Recently I had a patient ask if I was referring to 'neuroleptics' in inquiring about his drug history. Patients are becoming increasingly sophisticated, therefore, it behooves nurses to be better informed. . . . Incidentally, the question about neuroleptics came from a patient who one would describe as a 'street person.' He had no home and survived by literally sleeping in doorways."

It is your responsibility in nurse/patient interviews to continually check to make sure that you are accurately understanding the patient's perceptions and the patient is understanding your perceptions.

YOUR RESPONSIBILITIES IN NURSE/PATIENT INTERVIEWS

Not only do you in any nurse/patient interview have the responsibility of checking the accuracy of perceptions, but you also have many other responsibilities, some of which have already been discussed.

Before you actually conduct an interview with a patient/client, you have the responsibility of considering the general and specific purpose of the interview, the potential communication choices, and the possible results of these choices. You also have the responsibility of considering the potential nonverbal influences such as environment, and of preparing actual communicative strategies and types of questions to be asked.

During the conduct of the interview, you have the responsibility of beginning the interview, whenever possible, in a manner in which the social penetration process will not be violated. Also during the beginning of the interview, you should, whenever possible, explain precisely the purpose of the interview. By going through the ritual of the acquaintance process and explaining the purpose of the interview, you are likely to build rapport and trust with the patient and demonstrate empathy toward the patient. If these things occur, the chances for successful communication are increased.

In the body of the interview, you have the responsibility to continually monitor and assess communicative purposes, strategies, and outcomes. You must keep in mind that communicative success is most likely achieved when you exhibit CONSTANT ADAPTIVE BEHAVIOR.

In the close of a patient interview, you also have responsibilities. A nurse/patient interview is more likely to be successful if, during the close, you are consistent with what you have done previously in the interview, review and summarize for the patient what has been accomplished during the course of the interview, and explain to the patient what the patient can expect to happen next. Even though you may have all the information needed from a patient, the interview is not complete until the patient also has information—information about what has been accomplished in the interview and what is likely to occur next. If this conclusion is given by you, subsequent interviews with the patient are more likely to be successful. Finally, throughout the interview, *you* have the responsibility of checking perceptions.

So far in this chapter and in the previous chapter we have presented principles and theory and have placed many demands on you as interviewer—demands which we feel are essential if you are to be an effective communicator with patients. Let's attempt to apply these considerations to actual nurse/patient interviews.

CONDUCT AND ANALYSIS OF ACTUAL NURSE/PATIENT INTERVIEWS

Most writings in the area of nurse/patient communication are based upon the assumption that you can learn to be a good nursing communicator through "interaction" between you and the written words of the author. We seriously question this assumption. We believe you gain patient interviewing skills only through actual implementation of communication principles with patients. To become an effective communicator with patients, you must not only practice but you must also be able to understand and appreciate the beliefs, attitudes, values, and opinions of patients. These patient orientations are usually very different from your own.

One way for nurses to implement skills and to understand patient orientation is through role-playing. In the exercise that follows, you will be asked to role-play both nurse and patient. Through our experiences in workshops and in-services, we have found that optimal results are obtained when between three and twelve nurses are involved in the exercise. If more than twelve are involved, it is very difficult to conduct discussions in which everyone participates. The exercise is structured so that it can be used by you alone or with one other nurse, but you can gain maximum benefit if you participate in a small group.

In the exercise, you will be asked to conduct nursing rounds during a "typical" day in a "typical" hospital. During your rounds, you will encounter twelve patients who will test your interviewing skills.

If you are doing this exercise by yourself, you will play the nurse throughout. If two are participating, one of you, in the first situation, will play the nurse, the other will play the patient; you will alternate roles in subsequent situations. If three or more are involved, in the first situation, one person will play the nurse, one person the patient, one person will be a monitor, and all others will be observers who will say nothing before or during the interview. After the first situation, alternate roles so that through the course of the exercise, each participant has the opportunity to play nurse, patient, and monitor.

Each situation in the exercise begins with a configuration description, that is, a description of the patient, nursing orders relevant to the patient, and basic facts concerning the situation.

The first configuration description is preceded by a sample "pre-interview evaluation" form (Figure 9). On a separate sheet of paper, *the nurse is to use the format of Figure 9 to make an evaluation of the situation before the interview begins.* The same procedure is followed for each of the other eleven interviews.

Following the pre-interview evaluation form in the first interview exercise, an "observer interview evaluation" form (Figure 10, page 62) is given. This format is used in each interview to sketch how you think the interview would progress if you are doing the exercise by yourself, or used to evaluate the actual interview if a small group is involved in the exercise.

Finally each interview situation ends with a "patient orientation" description and "monitor/observer notes." If more than one person is involved in the exercise, each participant *except the nurse* will be familiar with the patient orientation; each participant *except nurse and patient* will be familiar with the monitor/observer notes.

For those of you doing the exercise by yourself, read the configuration and complete the pre-interview evaluation in the format of Figure 9. Next, using the format of Figure 10 as a guide, briefly sketch how you think the interview would progress. After you have completed these steps, read the patient orientation description and monitor/observer notes and make an assessment of how well you met the patient/situation demands *or* how well you could have adapted to these demands based upon your initial approach.

If only two nurses are involved in the exercise, both read the configuration description, the nurse completes the pre-interview evaluation form, the patient reads the patient orientation, the interview is conducted, both nurse and patient read the monitor/observer notes and discuss the interview according to the format of the observer interview evaluation.

When more than two nurses participate in the exercise, it is easiest to have the monitor read to everyone the configuration description and verbally ask the nurse the pre-interview analysis questions. The nurse writes answers to these questions on a separate sheet of paper but does *not* discuss these responses with anyone until *after* the interview has been completed.

After the nurse answers the pre-interview analysis questions, the monitor asks the nurse to leave the room. When the nurse is out of hearing distance, the monitor reads the patient orientation to the *patient* and the *observers*. The *monitor* and *observers silently* read the monitor/observer notes—the patient will *not* be familiar with these notes until *after* the interview. Having completed these tasks, the monitor calls the nurse to the room and the interview begins.

Time needed to complete each interview will vary. Some interviews

FIGURE 9 Nurse's Pre-Interview Evaluation

General purpose of interview (informative, persuasive, supportive):

Specific goal(s) in interview:

Interviewing strategies to achieve these goals and major advantages/disadvantages of each:

Strategy　　　　*Advantages*　　　　*Disadvantages*
Directive

Nondirective

Combination

Best alternative strategy considering the patient, the situation, and myself:

Most appropriate types of questions (open, direct, closed, yes/no, probes, restatements, mm-hm, silence, leading) to implement selected strategy:

Nonverbal communication factors important to situation:

FIGURE 10 Observer Interview Evaluation

During the interview, make notes on the right side of this form. Briefly write key questions, statements, and events that occur. After the interview, make a brief evaluation on the left side. Focus on the outline and issues listed.

Evaluative Comments   *List of actual questions, statements, events*

1. Opening:
   follows social penetration process,
   explains purpose

2. Body:
   type strategy used,
   logical sequencing

3. Closing:
   consistency, provides summary
   and future orientation

4. Overall:
   A. Checks accuracy of perceptions

   B. Questions:
      types used, appropriateness

   C. Statements:
      types used, appropriateness

   D. Accurately assesses problems,
      if any

will "naturally" come to a close. However, if the interview becomes too involved for time constraints or ceases to be productive, the monitor may end the interview at any point. Following the close of the interview, the monitor will lead the discussion based upon the pre-interview analysis made by the nurse and the comments of the observers made on the interview evaluation sheets.

A few general comments before you begin. We have found that the exercise is best accomplished if it is done in a setting that resembles a hospital room—a bed for the patient is particularly important. The more "real-life" the setting, the better. Also, try to have the observers in such a location that they are "observers" and not participants during the interview. Have the observers in a location where they can see and hear what is occurring, but such that they do not interfere with the interaction between nurse and patient during the interview.

During the conduct of the interviews, some of you may have a great deal of difficulty role-playing the patients as instructed. The lower your Rhetorical Sensitivity score (RS scale), the more difficulty you are likely to experience role-playing. However, it is essential for you and the others involved, to "place yourself in the patient's shoes," adopting and enacting the specified patient role for the situation. As you become more proficient in role-playing patients, you will be taking steps to personally become more Rhetorically Sensitive, and you will be providing experiences for the other participants to also increase their levels of Rhetorical Sensitivity. In these processes, you will all be taking steps to be more successful nurse communicators.

One other point we wish to stress: In no situation is there one right way or one wrong way to conduct the interview—there are many right and wrong ways. The purpose of the exericse is not to be perfect interviewers, but rather for all of you to learn. Let us put you to work.

NURSE/PATIENT INTERVIEWING EXERCISE

Interview #1   Configuration

The Patient: A 35-year-old female recovering from an episode of cholecystitis. A cholecystography has revealed no blockage of the bile duct and treatment is centered around modifications in diet.

Nursing Orders: Up ad lib. with rest period in morning and afternoon, observe for nausea, vomiting and/or epigastric distress, bland diet, begin diet instruction.

The Situation: It is 8 A.M. The patient's breakfast has been delivered and the food tray is sitting in front of her. The patient has made the comment to the nurse: "This food tastes awful."

Nurse's Pre-Interview Evaluation:
Use the format of Figure 9.

Observer Interview Evaluation:
Use the format of Figure 10.

Patient Orientation:
The patient is concerned about how to get her family of three school-age children and husband to go along with the special diet she must have. She doesn't see how she will have the energy to make separate meals for herself and also prepare meals for her family. In addition, the patient is feeling "old," "ugly," and "obese"—her weight has increased by twenty pounds in the past year. The patient will make statements such as: "This proves I'm getting old." "I'm just physically falling apart."

Monitor/Observer Notes:
This situation can usually best be handled by the nurse using a nondirective approach at least until all the patient's concerns are revealed. It is particularly important that the nurse allow the patient sufficient time to reveal her feelings—she has multiple concerns. Be particularly sensitive to questions/statements by the nurse that cut off the patient before she has fully expressed her feelings.

If the nurse does determine both the meal preparation and appearance concerns, does the nurse make any constructive comments relating the two such as how the recommended diet could possibly result in improved physical appearance? Also, be sensitive to comments by the nurse that downgrade the patient's feelings—statements such as, "That's not really important." Even though statements made by the patient could seem trivial to the nurse, they are not trivial to the patient.

The closing in this interview is very important, no matter what has been revealed during the interview. The nurse must give the patient a definite future orientation even if it is nothing more than, "I'll come back later and we can talk some more."

NURSE/PATIENT INTERVIEWING EXERCISE

Interview #2   Configuration

The Patient: A 29-year-old well-built, muscular male who is one day postoperative after a inguinal hernia repair. His scrotum is swollen, ecchymotic, and painful. Pain medication was last given at 10 PM the previous evening.

Nursing Orders: Regular diet, scrotum elevated when in bed and intermittent application of ice bag, wear jock strap when ambulatory, analgesics as required for pain.

The Situation: It is 8:30 AM. The patient is standing by a window and staring out the window.

Nurse's Pre-Interview Evaluation:
Use the format of Figure 9.

Observer Interview Evaluation:
Use the format of Figure 10.

Patient Orientation:
Even though the patient had preoperative teaching which included information about temporary physical changes to expect during the postoperative period, the patient is afraid the operation may have an adverse effect on his sex life. He is extremely reluctant to discuss these fears. He is in much pain but will *not* admit this to the nurse. However, during the interview, the pain will become so severe at times that he will have difficulty even speaking.

Monitor/Observer Notes:
In this situation, it will be essential for the nurse to get the patient away from the window—the nurse must attempt to get and maintain eye contact with the patient. The nurse may have to be very directive to accomplish this.

After the patient is away from the window, nondirective techniques offer the best chance of having the patient reveal his concerns. If and when the problem is revealed, the nurse must not show any signs of embarrassment or related emotions.

If the nurse is female (and especially if young and/or "uncomfortable"), one possible course of action that could be considered would be for the nurse to say, "If you would feel more comfortable discussing this with a male (nurse or physician), I'll be happy to get him to come talk to you."

Keep in mind that the pain may have an effect on the patient's verbalization of his feelings. When the pain is reduced, he may be better able and more willing to express his feelings. Does the nurse consider this factor?

NURSE/PATIENT INTERVIEWING EXERCISE

Interview #3   Configuration

The Patient: A 18-year-old female who has previously suffered face and neck burns and has been readmitted for reconstructive surgery.

Nursing Orders: Up ad lib, shower, nothing by mouth.

The Situation: It is 11 AM. At 1 PM, the patient is to undergo the first of several operations for reconstruction of facial and neck tissue.

A local television station recently broadcast a series on reconstructive surgery. In one show, an unsuccessful repair was reported in which infection occurred after surgery and further scarring developed. Both patient and nurse saw this show.

Nurse's Pre-Interview Evaluation:
Use the format of Figure 9.

Observer Interview Evaluation:
Use the format of Figure 10.

Patient Orientation:
The patient is very calm and very confident that the surgery will be successful.

Monitor/Observer Notes:
This situation requires the nurse be very supportive. The logical first impression by the nurse is that the patient is extremely apprehensive and scared. However, if the nurse attempts too hard to question the patient concerning fears or concern, the nurse is likely to create a problem where one did not exist before the interview.

Does the nurse overemphasize postoperative care and measures taken to prevent infection? Does the nurse make any remarks that might reduce the patient's confidence in the success of the procedure? Be particularly sensitive to questions by the nurse such as, "You're not scared at all? Not even a little bit?"

NURSE/PATIENT INTERVIEWING EXERCISE

Interview #4   Configuration

The Patient: A four-year-old male hospitalized with pneumonia.

Nursing Orders: Bed rest, liquid diet, complete bath.

The Situation: It is 2 PM—time for a routine check by the nurse. The child's parents are sitting in the room. The child is pouting—on the verge of crying.

Nurse's Pre-Interview Evaluation:
Use the format of Figure 9.

Observer Interview Evaluation:
Use the format of Figure 10.

Patient Orientation:
The boy wants his "rag doll" but has been told by his father that dolls are for sissies; they are not for "big boys." The father has just purchased a small football from the gift shop and given it to his son. (Two of the observers will role-play the child's parents and will be sitting in the room.)

Monitor/Observer Notes:
This can be an extremely difficult situation for the nurse. The nurse needs to listen to the child's feelings and be supportive of the child. However, the nurse cannot ignore the parents. The nurse must respect the parents' values and be careful not to downgrade them in front of the child.

To be successful requires the nurse, after discovering the child's feelings, talk to the parents *separately* from the child. The nurse must guard against talking to the parents in front of the child and acting as if the child was not present.

Also, when talking with the child, the nurse must use language that can be comprehended by the child on his level. Does the nurse talk with the child or does the nurse talk through the parents to the child? To be successful requires that the nurse talk with the child and on the child's level—respecting his individual needs and fears.

Another important aspect to consider is the child's developmental level. One child at this age may perceive a routine medical procedure as punishment while another child at the same age will take the procedure in stride. Does the nurse stereotype the child because of his age?

NURSE/PATIENT INTERVIEWING EXERCISE

Interview #5   Configuration

The Patient: A 75-year-old female who has suffered a cerebral vascular accident (CVA). The patient has severe paralysis on the left side and slurred speech. Previous to this illness, the patient lived on her own and cared for herself.

Nursing Orders: Transfer activity—bed to wheelchair, full weight bearing with assistance, soft diet.

The Situation: It is 5 PM. The patient has refused any offer of fluids during the past seven hours. The nurses have been kept busy throughout the day due to ward census and the many needs of patients.

Nurse's Pre-Interview Evaluation:
Use the format of Figure 9.

Observer Interview Evaluation:
Use the format of Figure 10.

Patient Orientation:
The patient is frustrated and angry. Nursing staff members have put the same dress on her for the past two days. Refusing to drink is a sign of protest, anger, and frustration.

Monitor/Observer Notes:
In this situation, or any situation in which a patient has lost functioning and abilities, it is important that the nurse provide a supportive atmosphere. The nurse needs to take the time to listen to the patient, allowing the patient to express her feelings in a relaxed and calm environment.

Since the patient's speech is impaired, does the nurse give the patient sufficient time to express her feelings? Is the nurse particularly sensitive to the patient's nonverbal cues? Nondirective techniques such as silence and restatements can be used to achieve beneficial results.

It is also important for the nurse to treat the patient as an intelligent adult. Does the nurse speak to the patient as an adult, or as if she were a child? If the patient feels the nurse sees her as a thinking adult, it becomes more likely that the interview will be constructive and successful.

Also consider nonverbal gestures of the nurse—does the nurse seem hurried and impatient?

NURSE/PATIENT INTERVIEWING EXERCISE

Interview #6   Configuration

The Patient: A 45-year-old male who is recovering from a recent myocardial infarction. The patient has a history of high blood pressure and is on antihypertensive drugs which have a tendency to cause periodic states of hypotension.

Nursing Orders: Bedside commode, up in chair 20 minutes q.i.d.

The Situation: It is 7:30 PM. Visiting hours are from 7 to 8:30 PM. The nurse discovers the patient pacing up and down the hospital corridor. It is snowing heavily outside.

Nurse's Pre-Interview Evaluation:
Use the format of Figure 9.

Observer Interview Evaluation:
Use the format of Figure 10.

Patient Orientation:
Patient is extremely concerned. His wife was supposed to visit this evening at the start of visiting hours but she has not yet arrived. Because of the snow storm, the patient is worried his wife may be stuck in the snow or involved in an accident. The patient's home is 35 miles from the hospital.

Monitor/Observer Notes:
In this situation, the nurse's primary concern must be for the patient's immediate safety. The nurse must be directive and get the patient back to bed or at least to a chair where he can sit. Time needed to employ nondirective techniques prohibits their use during the initial nurse/patient encounter in this situation.

Assuming the nurse has succeeded in getting the patient off his feet, does the nurse directly address the patient's concerns? The patient's condition and the need to alleviate any stressor events dictate immediate action by the nurse.

What type action does the nurse take? To begin, the nurse might try calling the patient's home to check if his wife had left for the hospital. If the nurse in the actual situation does this, the monitor will "answer the phone" and state: "She left home at 6:45 PM." In this case, there would be little cause for immediate concern and the patient should relax.

If the patient does not relax or if the nurse does *not* determine that the wife is not overdue, it may be necessary for the nurse to even check with police or highway patrol for accident reports. The nurse must take some action to lessen the patient's fear and to reassure him that his concerns are being actively considered.

The nurse could sit and wait with the patient until his wife finally arrives, or if this is not possible, find someone else to remain with the patient. The patient must be monitored closely until his concerns are resolved.

NURSE/PATIENT INTERVIEWING EXERCISE

Interview #7   Configuration

The Patient: A 22-year-old male recovering from a motorcycle accident. The patient suffered multiple fractures of the right femur. Patient is in traction which is applied by use of Thomas splint with Pearson attachment.

Nursing Orders: Bed rest, maintain pulley alignment with weights hanging freely, observe for skin irritation from traction bandages, circulatory checks every four hours.

The Situation: It is 10 PM. and the nurse is on routine rounds. It is time to take vital signs, do circulatory check, check traction, offer urinal.

Nurse's Pre-Interview Evaluation:
Use the format of Figure 9.

Observer Interview Evaluation:
Use the format of Figure 10.

Patient Orientation:
The patient is very attracted to the nurse and desires to have the nurse stay with him as long as possible. The patient will ask for water, a fresh pillow case, anything to keep the nurse in the room. The patient *must* get the nurse to stay in the room as long as possible.

Monitor/Observer Notes:
After the interview has become involved, the monitor will announce: "Down the hall, a patient's call bell is ringing. You (the nurse) are the only medical professional on the floor at this time." Note the communicative leave-taking techniques attempted by the nurse. What effect do these techniques have?

If the nurse does not respond to the call bell within two to three minutes, the monitor will end the interview by telling the nurse that the patient rang the call bell because the patient was having severe chest pains. This other patient had a myocardial infarction, and is now in cardiac arrest.

This obviously could be a very traumatic experience for the nurse, and is used to stress that the nurse has many responsibilities and must balance all concerns. This is a situation in which it is possible for the nurse to be too supportive to a particular patient and in the process jeopardize the welfare of other patients.

NURSE/PATIENT INTERVIEWING EXERCISE

Interview #8   Configuration

The Patient: A 22-year-old male recovering from a motorcycle accident. This patient is a friend of the patient in Interview #7 and was involved in the

70 Communicating with Patients

same accident. This patient also has a fractured right femur and is in traction.

Nursing Orders: Bed rest, maintain pulley alignment with weights hanging freely, observe for skin irritation from traction bandages, circulatory checks every four hours.

The Situation: It is 10:30 PM and the nurse is continuing routine rounds after the incident in Interview #7. The nurse must take vital signs, do circulatory check, check traction, offer urinal.

Nurse's Pre-Interview Evaluation:
Use the format of Figure 9.

Observer Interview Evaluation:
Use the format of Figure 10.

Patient Orientation:
The patient will inform the nurse that his right leg feels slightly uncomfortable. The patient will have *no other* special problems, concerns, desires, etc.

Monitor/Observer Notes:
In this situation it is likely that the nurse will be extremely cautious because of experiences with the previous patient. How much does the nurse carry over feelings from the previous patient?

If the nurse stereotypes from the previous patient, the nurse is likely to exhibit defensive behavior toward this patient. Does the nurse hurry through the tasks and only "half listen" to what the patient says? Observe any nonverbal signs of defensiveness by the nurse such as prolonged standing at a social-consultative distance (4 to 12 feet) from the patient, and assuming a defensive body position with arms crossed in front of the nurse's body. Also, observe for defensiveness in the nurse's verbal statements and questions to the patient.

How do the actions of the nurse affect the patient and how do these actions influence patient care?

In this situation, we have attempted to stress that each patient is unique and must be treated as a separate individual with specific health care needs. Do the nurse's communicative actions accomplish this goal?

NURSE/PATIENT INTERVIEWING EXERCISE

Interview #9   Configuration

The Patient: A 30-year-old female who is second day postpartum after delivering her fifth baby. The baby boy weighs eight pounds nine ounces and is doing well. Mother and baby are scheduled to be discharged in the morning.

Nursing Orders: Up ad lib.; self-care; regular diet; discharge teaching to include breast care, involutional changes, activity, family planning, and signs and symptoms to report to physician; baby care instruction.

The Situation: It is 12:30 AM. The patient cannot get to sleep. She was given a sleeping pill at 10 PM but is still awake.

Nurse's Pre-Interview Evaluation:
Use the format of Figure 9.

Observer Interview Evaluation:
Use the format of Figure 10.

Patient Orientation:
Three of the patient's five children are under school age. Her husband is a salesman and away from home most of the week. She feels very tired because of the demands made upon her by so many young children. Her husband is taking two weeks' vacation to help out at home but then will be returning to work—leaving her with most of the responsibility for total child care.

The patient does not want any more children. She wants a tubal ligation, however has not expressed this to anyone because of religious beliefs. The patient will attempt to get the nurse to make the decision for her having the tubal ligation.

Monitor/Observer Notes:
In this situation, the greatest chance of success is for the nurse to use a nondirective approach throughout the interview. The nurse *cannot* make decisions for the patient. If the nurse makes the patient's decision and any problems, conflicts, etc., develop afterward, the patient is likely to view the nurse as the cause of difficulty.

Does the nurse inform the patient of hospital regulations for tubal ligations? If the nurse does not know the regulations, does the nurse indicate a willingness to find out for the patient? Does the nurse inform the patient of alternatives for family planning? If so, does the nurse do this in an objective manner? Does the nurse succeed in having the patient take responsibility for decision making?

NURSE/PATIENT INTERVIEWING EXERCISE

Interview #10   Configuration

The Patient: A 55-year-old male who is hospitalized for two days for his annual physical and routine laboratory tests. This examination is required by his place of employment.

Nursing Orders: Regular diet, up ad lib.

The Situation: It is 1 AM. The patient checked into the hospital seven hours earlier. The patient is awake and has the light on above his bed. He is reading a business magazine.

Nurse's Pre-Interview Evaluation:
Use the format of Figure 9.

Observer Interview Evaluation:
Use the format of Figure 10.

Patient Orientation:
The patient is slightly apprehensive about his tests tomorrow, but not overly concerned. The patient is not tired; his normal bedtime is 2 AM—the patient will *not* tell the nurse his usual bedtime *unless directly asked* by the nurse.

Monitor/Observer Notes:
In this situation, if the nurse uses a combination approach, the nurse should be able to easily discover that there really is no problem or concern from the patient's standpoint. It is simply not time for the patient to go to sleep.

If the nurse uses a very directive approach throughout the interview, the nurse is unlikely to discover the proper facts, for it is unlikely to think to ask, "What is your usual bedtime?"

If the nurse uses a straight nondirective approach, the nurse is also unlikely to discover the proper facts because of the patient orientation (as specified by the instructions to patient). However, by mixing nondirective and directive techniques, the nurse should have little problem in discovering the facts.

NURSE/PATIENT INTERVIEWING EXERCISE

Interview #11   Configuration

The Patient: A 16-year-old female who is two days postpartum after delivery of a premature infant. The patient is unmarried and this is her first child. The baby is in the neonatal intensive care unit and is receiving oxygen via oxyhood. The mother is recovering satisfactorily. The baby's condition has been stable for the last 24 hours.

Nursing Orders: Routine postpartum care, assess home support system, allow patient time to express feelings.

The Situation: It is 5 AM. The mother is awake and rings the call bell.

Nurse's Pre-Interview Evaluation:
Use the format of Figure 9.

Observer Interview Evaluation:
Use the format of Figure 10.

Patient Orientation:
The mother would like to see her baby. She not only wants to see the baby, but also wants to hold the baby *and* have the baby in the room with her. The mother will be very insistent that her requests be honored.

Monitor/Observer Notes:
In this situation, the nurse needs to be both firm and supportive. For many young mothers, labor and delivery are frightening experiences; and even though they are told their infants are all right, it is difficult for them to believe.

Obviously, the nurse cannot fulfill all the mother's demands. However, the nurse can reassure the mother and make arrangements for the mother to see and possibly hold the baby in the neonatal intensive care unit.

Be particularly sensitive to whether the nurse gives adequate explanations why some of the mother's requests cannot be met. If the nurse does not try to explain reasons to the mother, and/or if the nurse becomes too forceful in reaction to the mother's demands, the mother may react in a negative manner becoming even more insistent and upset.

It is important for the nurse to respect both the needs of the mother and the hospital and medical policies in this situation.

NURSE/PATIENT INTERVIEWING EXERCISE

Interview #12   Configuration

The Patient: A 55-year-old female who has had a nonmalignant mass removed from her breast. The patient is to be released from the hospital the following day.

Nursing Orders: Regular diet, shower, up ad lib.

The Situation: It is 6 AM. and the patient is awake. The patient has asked the nurse for a cup of coffee. The nurse is returning with the coffee.

Nurse's Pre-Interview Evaluation:
Use the format of Figure 9.

Observer Interview Evaluation:
Use the format of Figure 10.

Patient Orientation:
After the patient receives the coffee, she will start "small talk" with the nurse. The patient will then ask the nurse to read to her everything on her medical chart.

The patient believes she has cancer even though her mass was determined to be benign. Two of her closest friends have recently been diagnosed as having cancer; one is scheduled for surgery in two days.

Each time the nurse makes a statement about the patient's condition, the patient will state: "That means I have cancer, doesn't it?"

Monitor/Observer Notes:
In this situation, the patient has legal rights to certain information. However, the nurse is responsible for reporting only information to which the nurse has accountability and that the nurse knows to be factual.

In reporting any type information to the patient, it is important not only that the information is accurate, but that the patient's perceptions of the information are also accurate. It is therefore important for the nurse to assess the patient's understanding of the condition already known and her general understanding of medical information.

In the situation given, if the nurse simply answers "No" each time the patient says, "That means I have cancer..." it is unlikely the patient's perceptions will change or be any more accurate than they were before the interview.

Observe if the nurse gives explanations and reasons behind the "no" responses. These explanations should be maintained within legal and ethical boundaries of health care practice.

Finally, it is important for the nurse to explore the patient's fears concerning cancer and help to alleviate these concerns before the patient is released from the hospital. If the nurse does not have the knowledge necessary to interpret the medical information, the nurse should explain this to the patient and find someone who can answer the patient's questions.

This exercise has been designed not as an end point but rather as a starting point. Through participating in the exercise, we hope that you have gained some insight into what it means for you to become more Rhetorically Sensitive. It means that you must treat each patient/client and each situation as unique. In each interaction with a patient/client, you must consider the multitude of communicative choices available; you must carefully weigh the potential outcomes of enacting these various choices; you must exhibit constant adaptive behavior; you must select communicative choices that serve the needs of the patient/client and the situation but also serve your own needs and maintain your integrity.

Progress in your becoming more successful nurse communicators can only be made by your taking what you have experienced and learned and applying it daily in your communicative encounters. You will never be perfect communicators, but you must constantly strive for this unattainable goal. It will only be through such striving that you will become more successful.

SUMMARY

In this chapter, we have identified your main communicative function as interaction with patients/clients. We have stressed the uniqueness of each of you, each patient you encounter, and each situation involving a patient. In addition, we have attempted to impress that there are no right or wrong answers to any communicative question—in each communicative encounter there are many right ways to attain a goal, just as there are many ways not to attain the goal.

We have placed focus on your responsibilities in interviews with patients/clients. You have responsibility to adequately prepare for each interview. You have responsibility at the start of each interview to enact an orderly social penetration process if possible. You have responsibility during each interview to understand and check perceptions, meta perceptions, etc. made by both you and the patient. You have responsibility at the close of each interview to ensure that not only you but also the patient understands what has been accomplished and what will occur next.

Finally, we have attempted to make the concerns, considerations, and principles discussed so far become a part of you through your participation in a nurse/patient interviewing exercise.

In the remaining chapters of this book, you should take what you have learned and expand this knowledge by applying it to other significant nursing communicative configurations—configurations involving nonpatient others.

References

Altman, I., & Taylor, D. A. *Social penetration: The development of interpersonal relationships.* New York: Holt, Rinehart and Winston, Inc., 1973.

Laing, R. D., Phillipson, H., & Lee, A. R. *Interpersonal perception.* New York: Springer Publishing Company, 1966.

Searight, R. Being honest with Gary was the least—and the most—we could do. *Nursing 80,* February 1980, 55-56.

Suggested Readings

Benjamin, A. *The helping interview* (3rd ed.). Boston: Houghton Mifflin Company, 1981.
Focuses on interviewing as a process for developing relationships characterized by mutual trust and creative change. Provides provocative discussion of interviewing techniques whenever interviews are used as methods for providing support.

Nursing Times. 1981.
A major weekly nursing journal of Great Britain.

The *Nursing Times* (NT) declared 1981 the year of communication. As part of the NT's coverage of communication, many issues throughout the year contained articles relating to communication skills.

Of particular note were 24 articles labeled "Talking Points" which were published on an almost weekly basis from January 29, to July 29, 1981. Each "Talking Point" contained an actual transcript of a nurse/patient interaction, and discussion of communication problems and techniques associated with the interaction.

CHAPTER 4

Communicating with Health Care Professionals

Although we consider the nurse's primary communicative responsibility to be interviews with patients, as a nurse you have other major communicative demands. You must function as a member of a total health care team; you must communicate with superiors, peers, and subordinates both within nursing and outside nursing; and you must, at times, communicate with the general public.

In this chapter we shall discuss interviews with nursing colleagues, physicians, and other health care team members, and we shall discuss you as communicator in small groups with these other health care professionals—a small group defined as consisting of 3 to 12 people engaged in a mutual communicative experience.

NONPATIENT NURSING INTERVIEWS

Not only must you communicate in one-to-one situations with patients, but you must also communicate in one-to-one situations with other nurses, physicians, and other health care team members. Considerations and principles presented in the previous chapters *all* apply to interviews with health care colleagues. In other words, in colleague interviews, you must analyze the situation and communicative demands; plan the interview as much as possible; employ sound interviewing practices such as appropriate strategies and questions; balance your self-concerns with the concerns of the other; and exhibit constant adaptive behavior.

However, in such interviews there is one factor that often overrides all other factors. Whenever patient health care issues are involved, patient well-being supersedes all other concerns even if it means jeopardizing nurse/colleague relationships and participants' individual desires and needs. Consider the following actual examples provided by two of our nurse respondents (names have been changed).

SITUATION   A maternity patient is in the postpartum recovery room. It is 11 PM on a Saturday evening. The patient had delivered her baby (her third child) at 10 PM. The attending physician has left the hospital and is now at home. The maternity nurse in charge calls the physician at his home. Their conversation is as follows:

NURSE: Dr. Long, Mrs. Hendrick's blood pressure is 100/60 and her pulse is 84. When she was admitted to the recovery room BP was 116/74, pulse 60. Her fundus is firm and the external vaginal bleeding is moderate. I think she may be bleeding internally but I'm not sure because there's no excessive external vaginal bleeding. I'm particularly concerned because she's become restless and I'm just not comfortable with her behavior.

DOCTOR: Okay, just watch her.

NURSE: I feel the patient needs to be evaluated by a physician. The only physician here is Dr. Bradley and he just went into the delivery room with another patient.

DOCTOR: Okay, just watch her and call me back if there's any further change.

NURSE: But doctor, I think she needs to be evaluated now.

DOCTOR: I told you to just watch her and . . .

NURSE: I'm telling you to get in here because there is something wrong, and I don't know what it is.

DOCTOR: Okay, okay, I'll come in. I'm sure it's nothing very important.

SITUATION   A male patient has had major abdominal surgery. The patient is one day postoperative and in the med/surg ward of a small rural hospital. The patient is being monitored by a staff nurse for possible hemorrhage. Blood has been typed and cross-matched and blood is ready in the blood bank. It is 2 PM. The physician had checked the patient at 1 PM and is now in the hospital clinic which is one floor below and at the opposite end of the building from the med/surg ward. The staff nurse phones the physician. Their conversation is as follows:

NURSE: Doctor, Mr. Coyle's BP is down to 86/40. Pulse is 110 and thready.

DOCTOR: I was afraid of this. Prepare him for a return to surgery. You stay with the patient and send someone to get the blood from the lab and I'll be right up to start it. We don't have any time to waste.

The nurse goes to the nurse's station where a nurse's aide is sitting on a chair with her feet propped up on another chair. The conversation between the nurse and the aide is as follows:

NURSE: Ms. Booth, go to the lab and get blood for Mr. Coyle—he has to have emergency surgery.

AIDE: No!

NURSE: Why?

AIDE: Because I don't like the way you talked to me.

The nurse grasps the aide by the arm and pulls her to an adjacent hallway away from patient rooms. The conversation continues.

NURSE: The patient needs blood now, this is serious.

AIDE: I don't like the way you asked me so I'm not going.

NURSE: I'm ordering you to go to the lab now! I don't care what you think of me, but you better be concerned about the welfare of that patient who needs blood now! So, go!

With that, the nurse pushes the aide toward the doorway leading to the lab.

Communicative disasters? By no means, for in both cases patients are alive who otherwise might have died.

In the first example of the maternity patient, the doctor arrived at the hospital by 11:15 PM and before midnight he had taken the patient to surgery for a repair of a tear at the junction of the uterus and fallopian tube.

In the second example of the med/surg patient, the aide got the blood and arrived with it at the patient's room at about the same time as the physician arrived. The patient was immediately taken to surgery where the hemorrhage was stopped and the patient recovered.

There are several similarities in these examples. Both examples involve patients with serious internal bleeding, even though the medical facts presented in the interviews clearly indicate the seriousness of the problem in the second case but not in the first.

If the situations are analyzed from the standpoint of nurse/colleague interaction, both nurses appear to violate interviewing principles we have discussed. Each nurse appears to be a Noble Self by being intolerant of a colleague's desires, showing little concern for the perceptions or needs of the colleague, and disregarding potential negative effects in terms of future relationship with the colleague.

However, if the interviews are analyzed from the standpoint of patient well-being, each nurse is Rhetorically Sensitive and each nurse enacts interviewing principles we have discussed. Each nurse assumes the role of interviewer even though the maternity nurse is in a role subordinate position (in reference to the physician) and the med/surg nurse is in a role superior position (in reference to the aide). Each nurse attempts to only communicate reports—vital signs and observations of behavior in the first example; sound professional medical judgments in the second example. Each nurse recognizes that the interviewee does not perceive the statements as reports but rather as inferences or possibly judgments. Each nurse attempts to clarify these statements. But, when the interviewee does not readily change perceptions, the nurse, because of facts and professional judgments relating to the patient, acts and chooses the best available communicative alternative for ensuring patient well-being.

You might ask, if the maternity patient in the first example did not have a serious problem, would the nurse still be considered Rhetorically Sensitive? Yes, because the nurse considered medical facts, experience, and professional judgment and chose the alternative that was safest for the most significant person involved, the patient. The nurse took a personal risk, but in so doing, minimized the risk for the patient. To be willing to take personal risks if "success" in the overall communicative configuration can be obtained is to be Rhetorically Sensitive.

In this discussion, we are not suggesting that you always appear as a Noble Self to non-nursing colleagues, or that these people always need to be told what to do. All that we are advocating is that the professionalism of nursing requires you enter most interactions with medical colleagues willing to take on the role of interviewer, and that whenever patient considerations are involved, the patient's needs must come before any other needs.

It was stressed that in most nursing interview situations, you should consider yourself the interviewer. But what if two nurses are involved in the interview? Can both take on the role of the interviewer?

Interviews with Nursing Peers, Subordinates, and Superiors

In situations involving patient information, not only can two nurses in an interview be interviewers, but they should both be interviewers if they desire the greatest chance of communicative success. That is, they should both assume the responsibilities of interviewer and seek information, clarification, and understanding to provide better patient care.

In some situations, however, especially situations involving performance appraisal or reprimand, only one person can assume the primary responsibilities of interviewer—the nurse giving the appraisal or reprimand. This does not mean that during the course of such interviews, interviewer/interviewee roles cannot alternate, but such reversals should only be of short duration.

When we asked our nurse respondents what types of communication problems they encountered with nursing peers, subordinates, and superiors, the most common problem reported involved situations in which the nurse must reprimand a subordinate for a mistake, omission, or inappropriate behavior or the nurse must appraise a subordinate's performance when that performance is less than satisfactory. Most of us have little difficulty communicating to a person positive aspects about that person, but when it comes to communicating aspects that may be perceived as negative, it is a different story.

How to Conduct Nursing Reprimands and Appraisals. The first guideline for successful communication in nursing reprimands or appraisals is that such situations should be dealt with in a direct face-to-face manner. In such high risk, tension packed situations, many of us attempt to avoid direct face-to-face interaction. For example, it is less threatening for the interviewer to write out a negative appraisal (or simply check boxes on a standard form) and hand it to the interviewee in a sealed envelope, or better yet, to send it by mail. While avoiding face-to-face interaction, such tactics do allow communication—nonpersonal communication that can create distrust, resentment, and feeling to avoid direct face-to-face interaction in the future. Only through face-to-face interaction in such situations can the nurse even hope to be an effective communicator. Face-to-face interaction allows individual perceptions to be checked, extenuating circumstances to be discussed, and/or mutually satisfying solutions to be developed. Not that these results are guaranteed, but at least, in face-to-face interaction, these outcomes are a possibility.

Once in a face-to-face reprimand or appraisal situation, what can you as interviewer do? Perhaps the most important interviewing issue in reprimands or appraisals involves the interviewer's use of statements.

You, as interviewer, should restrict, as much as possible, all of your statements to reports as opposed to inferences or judgments.

Assume that you are a staff nurse called in for a conference with your supervisor. Your supervisor makes the statement, "You're doing a bad job." How would you react? Would you be angry? Would you be defensive? Just what would you feel and how would you act? It is safe to assume you would have some kind of negative feelings toward your supervisor, and it is also safe to assume that the chances for this interview to be constructive and "successful" are slim. What type of statement did the supervisor make? The statement was a judgment, and as we have previously discussed, judgments stop thought processes and severely hinder any chance for effective communication.

Now consider the same circumstances, except that the supervisor states, "Because of med errors, your performance is unsatisfactory." In this situation, how would you react?

We will assume med errors were a fact—they did occur. However, in the supervisor's statement, the supervisor inferred you were the person responsible for the errors. If the supervisor's inference was correct, the interview could satisfactorily proceed even though it would likely be a very stressful situation for both parties. But, what if the supervisor's inference was not correct? You were not responsible for the med errors. How would you react? You would probably be very angry and defensive, and the remainder of the interview would likely be negatively influenced by these feelings.

Inferences allow the potential for misinterpretation. If misinterpretation occurs during an interview, the chance for successful interview completion decreases. Emotions and ill feelings are often aroused by misinterpretations, and once these factors are present, they are very difficult to control.

Inferences make the job of effective communication very difficult and if treated as fact and nonverified can result in inappropriate action taking place. In our situation, if you had not made the med errors, to be reprimanded by your superior would be very inappropriate.

Now consider the same situation except your supervisor begins by making the statement, "Last week, while you were on duty, there were three med errors." How would you react to this statement?

This statement contains no explicit inferences or judgments. The statement, by itself, is a report—a fact capable of verification. While the situation is still emotionally charged and implicit inferences and judgments could be made, the statement, by itself, does allow you, as interviewee, to explain your perceptions in a more objective manner than either previous situation. If, in fact, the med errors were not your fault, this could be determined without creating many of the ill feelings that would result if the interview had begun with an inference or judgment by the interviewer.

In addition to communicating in terms of reports as much as possible, when you conduct reprimands or appraisals you should be particularly cautious of two other factors. The first of these deals with the use of threats. Threats should be avoided as much as possible, and only used as a last resort when all else has failed. In addition, if a threat is used, you must be willing and able to carry out that threat if necessary. For example, if you have on several occasions reprimanded a subordinate for a particular unacceptable behavior and the behavior persists and concerns a serious matter such as patient well-being, you may find it necessary to use a threat such as, "If this behavior continues, you will be fired." However, you must have the power to fire the person and must be willing, if necessary, to do so. We must stress again that threats should be used only as a last alternative when no other choice exists.

One final caution concerns demonstrations of anger. In situations such as reprimands, feelings of anger by both the interviewer and interviewee are very common. In such circumstances, if you hope to be a successful communicator, you must avoid any demonstration of anger. This avoidance is extremely difficult but necessary if you are to remain in control of the situation—a natural inclination is to respond to anger with anger; if someone yells at us we tend to yell back. However, for you to be successful, you should remain in control of your emotions and the interview.

The communication issues involved when you interact with a nursing superior are similar to the issues involved when interacting with nursing peers and subordinates. When communicating with nursing superiors, you often can, and should, function as an interviewer. However, there are times when you must be the interviewee.

The Nurse as Interviewee. Many characteristics of a successful interviewee are the same as characteristics of a successful interviewer. If you are a competent nurse interviewee, you are able to listen both to what is being said and how it is being said. You are able to constantly adapt throughout the interview, employ appropriate strategies, continually check perceptions, clarify issues through the use of proper questioning techniques, refrain from threats, and control inclinations toward anger.

As an interviewee you plan and prepare for the interview. Preparation to be a nurse interviewee involves obtaining as much information, preferably in the form of reports, as possible so that accurate, complete answers to interview questions may be given. As nurse interviewer you prepare questions; as nurse interviewee you prepare answers. You should keep in mind that if you are an interviewee, during the course of the interview, you may assume the role of interviewer if needed to better fulfill interview objectives.

In summary, when communicating with other nurses in interview situations, you should employ the same basic principles and techniques employed in patient interviews.

Communicating with Physicians

Few topics in nursing spark as much controversy as communication between nurses and physicians. Traditionally, many have assumed the nurse's job in communicating with physicians was to passively listen, not to question, and faithfully obey the communicative dictates of a physician. The physician was the INTERVIEWER; the nurse was the nonresistant interviewee. While few nurses would openly advocate such a view today, many people outside the nursing field still cling to this archaic belief. It is our position that, if you are to be a successful nurse communicator, you must be willing to assume the role of active interviewer in interactions with physicians. We will explore what this position means by first presenting a few typical statements concerning nurse/physician communication made by our nurse respondents. The question was asked of our respondents, "When communicating with physicians, what types of communication problems do you encounter?" Following are typical answers that were received.

> In most situations I've had excellent communication with the physicians, however, sometimes it hasn't been quite as good. I think the more professionally competent the physician thinks you are, the better the situation in terms of communication. But I also think you need to be honest with physicians and let them know where you're coming from and what your ideas are. And if you disagree with them, just tell them that you disagree to their face without discussing it with somebody else. I have to admit though, this is easier to do with a physician you've worked with a lot as opposed to working with someone for the first time.

> I guess the major problem would be in communicating that I, in fact, can make observations to communicate to them accurately. That my observations are accurate and they can make some sort of a decision based upon my observations.

> When I do have problems, the most frequent problem seems to be the physician who does not listen to what the nurse has to say. He already has made up his mind how certain patients have to be cared for and trying to get the physician to elaborate on his position is difficult. That's where I think I encounter most of my communication problems.

The nurse and physician must mutually communicate if an outcome of proper patient care is desired. What does this mean? Does it mean that you should consider yourself an equal with the physician? Yes and no. Both you and the physician should share equally in responsibilities as communicators, but each of you has distinct medical (and legal) responsibilities. You are not a mini-physician; you are a nurse with nursing responsibilities to fulfill. Nurses and physicians should not view themselves as competitors but rather as cooperative partners in providing quality health care.

You should carry out a physician's orders concerning medication and medical procedures. But what if you, based on your professional judgment and/or knowledge concerning an individual patient, disagree with these orders as did the maternity nurse in the example at the beginning of this chapter?

How should you communicate this concern to the physician? Note that we did not say "Should you communicate this concern..." but rather "How should you communicate this concern . . ."

During the past decade countless programs, seminars, and workshops have been developed that claim, either directly or indirectly, to give you the answer to this question and also make you a better person (for a small fee, of course). One example of such attempts falls under the heading "assertiveness training." In many assertiveness training programs, or similar programs, nurses are told that they must believe in themselves and express their true feelings especially when attempting to communicate with physicians. While for some nurses, such training may make them better communicators with physicians, for many more nurses, in our opinion, such training hinders effective communication because of at least two important reasons.

First, most training programs are conducted in very artificial environments. This means that all participants are taught the same things and tend to develop common attitudes and beliefs. Under such conditions, certain communicative techniques can work very well, however, outside these sterile conditions, people do not hold the same attitudes and beliefs, and techniques may, and often do, have very different outcomes. Second, while most devotees of such training state that there is a difference between assertive behavior and aggressive behavior, few people, from our experience, are able to make this distinction in actual practice.

Let's return to the original question concerning how you should communicate legitimate concerns to a physician, and, in the process, discuss the distinction between being assertive and being aggressive.

A nurse should be assertive in communicating with a physician. How can we make this statement when it was just stated that assertiveness training usually doesn't work? We can state you must be assertive because assertive can be defined as meaning that you control yourself and the immediate environment, but do *not* control the other person. Attempts to control the other person can be defined as aggressive behavior or manipulative behavior.

How can you, when you have legitimate concerns that need to be expressed to a physician, be assertive but not aggressive or manipulative? You can be assertive by being Rhetorically Sensitive, that is, assuming the role of interviewer, accepting the responsibilities of interviewer, and conducting an interview in accord with the principles we have detailed.

Communicating with Other Health Care Team Members

When you interact with administrators, directors, planners, educators, therapists, technicians, and other health care team members on a one-to-one basis, the interviewing principles and practices discussed so far need also be implemented if you are to be a successful communicator. Communicating with other health care team members is basically the same as communicating with other nurses or with physicians.

Our nursing respondents identified two major areas that they felt were particularly important communicative concerns when interacting with non-nursing, non-physician health care team members—clarifying role relationships and clarifying terminology used in actual language. For example, one nurse described general role problems as follows:

> I think the main thing is understanding where they are coming from with some of their information, their techniques, what we can expect from them, what they expect of us—this type of thing. They have to know what our role and capabilities are, and we have to know what theirs are.

Another nurse offered the following narrative of a specific role problem she had encountered:

> Recently I made the mistake of telling a patient that because I was a nurse, I would not be engaging in a certain activity with him. The patient had made an inappropriate sexual request of me. The nurses' aides, male and female, were very offended. The feeling was that I had flaunted my status and implied that the patient's approaches would have been all right with other female staff members but not nurses! Certainly that was not what I intended to communicate.

Another nurse clearly identified the problem of language:

> I guess probably my main problem is using terminology that they can understand, and having them use terminology I can understand. People in different areas of health care tend to develop their own vocabularies. We seem to get in the habit of using certain phrases, words, abbreviations that people in the same area will understand, but we have to be careful that people in other areas, with different backgrounds, can also understand us.

In all interactions, but especially in interviews with non-nursing, non-physician health care team members, you, as a nurse, have a responsibility to ensure accurate role understanding. You also have a responsibility to ensure understanding and accurate use of terminology. Note that we have placed the responsibility on you, not the other.

So far in the book we have focused on the nurse as communicator in two-party interactions. While most communicative situations in nursing involve two parties, they are not the only communicative situations with which you must deal.

NURSING SMALL GROUP COMMUNICATION

Nurses also have to interact as members of small groups. As stated earlier, a small group will be defined simply as 3 to 12 people mutually interacting to achieve some overall goal.

You are involved in many different types of small groups formed for many different purposes. Our nursing respondents identified a wide variety of small groups in which they had participated ranging from routine nursing meetings at shift change, to counseling situations involving patients and patients' families, to major problem-solving groups consisting of professionals from many disciplines.

The composition of these small groups can vary greatly, such as being all nurses; nurses, physicians and/or health care team members; nurses and patients; or nurses and patient families. The purpose of the groups can also vary greatly. For example, small groups may be formed to solve problems, coordinate efforts, plan for the future, or simply to seek information, just to name a few examples.

On a sheet of paper, using the format supplied in Figure 11, list examples of small groups that you have recently participated in as part of your nursing duties. For now, simply list the purpose of the group and briefly describe the type of participants.

The dynamics of small group interaction, in many respects, are even more complex than the dynamics of two-party interaction. In small groups, two-party interactions are present between continually changing sets of participants. In addition, various unique phenomena occur simply because of the group. To describe these small group complexities, let's begin by asking the question: We have stressed the roles and responsibilities of the nurse as interviewer in two-party interactions, but what are your roles and responsibilities as a member of a small group?

Return to your Nursing Small Group Log. Next to each situation you have listed, briefly write what you perceive your role and your responsibilities were in that group. Also mark each situation on a scale of 1 to 10 in terms of how successful the group was in terms of achieving

FIGURE 11 Nursing Small Group Log

Purpose of Group	Type Participants	Role and Responsibilities	Rating 1 to 10	Group Leader

the overall goal you listed—a marking of 10 would be very successful, 5 moderately successful, 1 unsuccessful, etc.

If you listed several groups in your Log, you probably found yourself listing a variety of purposes, roles, and responsibilities. Some of these items were probably very easy to specify, others very difficult. Did you find that your success ratings for those groups for which it was easy to specify purpose, role, and responsibility (no matter what they were) were higher than your success ratings of those groups for which you had difficulty completing the table? Normally small groups are more successful in terms of final outcome when the purpose of the group is clearly understood, and roles and responsibilities of the members are defined. Specifying purpose, roles, and responsibilities implies *organization* which is prerequisite for successful communication within a small group.

Small Group Leadership and Leaders

How is organization achieved in a small group? Perhaps the primary method is through *leadership*. Small groups, to be successful, need to be organized and to be organized they need some form of leadership structure. Return to your Log. For each group you have listed, specify the leader in that group.

For those groups in which it was easy to specify a leader, were your ratings of success high or low? In most cases, the ratings were probably high, however, in some cases the ratings may have been low. Low ratings could result because there is a distinction between leader and leadership.

Leaders can be appointed or designated because of role position, subject matter expertise or any one of countless criteria. However, just because a person is specified as being a formal group leader does not mean that that person can supply leadership. John Brilhart (1978) has described the characteristics of effective discussion leaders (that is, small group leaders who provide leadership) as follows:

Effective leaders:

- have a good grasp of the problem (or task) facing the group
- are skilled in organizing group thinking
- are active in participation
- speak well
- are open minded
- are democratic and consultative
- have respect for and sensitivity to others
- can take on distinctive roles
- share rewards and give credit to the group

If you are designated leader of a group, to be an effective communicator you must keep in mind and demonstrate these small group leadership characteristics. You will note these characteristics are not all that different from the characteristics that were described for an effective interviewer.

What if you are not the formal group leader, but the designated leader does not demonstrate leadership? Should you simply allow the group to fail? Of course not, for you can, and, in our opinion, have the responsibility to assume leadership.

If you are in a small group leadership position, either formal or informal, you should demonstrate the characteristics of an effective leader that are listed above. In addition, Professor Brilhart offers the following guidelines for actually organizing and leading group discussion:

- always establish a cooperative group goal
- give praise, when deserved, to the group, not individuals
- keep the focus on common experience
- limit the number of issues or topics
- plan a variety of open-ended questions
- be guided by the nature of the subject
- focus on how the subject relates to interests of the members of the group

Enacting these principles increases the chances of group success, but does not ensure such success. Among many small group phenomena that can influence group effectiveness and success are groupthink, hidden agenda, norms, and cohesiveness.

Groupthink

Irving Janis (1973) has described a phenomenon that he calls *groupthink* that can dramatically influence group functioning and decisions, usually in a negative manner. Groupthink refers to a tendency for a member of a group to conform to a belief expressed by a prominent member of the group or a majority of the group even if such belief is contrary to the personal belief of the individual.

An example of groupthink given by one of our nurse respondents is as follows:

> We had a group that was formed to try to find out if there was any reason for a recent increase in infections on our ward. The group consisted of a physician and five nurses. During a meeting that we had, the physician stated what he thought the problem was and we all said we agreed. After the meeting, when just the nurses were talking with each other, we found out all of us really disagreed with the physician. But none of us, in the meeting, were willing to disagree with him, I guess, just because he was the physician.

To be successful communicators in small groups, nurses, whether in leadership positions or not, must continually assess statements made in the group and question members of the group whenever there is an indication that groupthink is occurring.

DISCUSSION QUESTION

Can you think of a small group that you were a member of in which groupthink occurred? What were the outcomes of that group?

Hidden Agenda

Another phenomenon in small groups that can have negative impact on group functioning and decisions is labeled *hidden agenda*. A hidden agenda occurs when an individual or subgroup within a group has an objective unexpressed to other group members which is different from the avowed group purpose.

One of our nurse respondents gave us the following example of a hidden agenda:

> The director of nursing calls weekly head nurses' meetings in which all the head nurses come and discuss with each other and with her, problems we may have had, and, just in general how things are going in our areas. A month ago, the assistant nursing director resigned to take another job, and word has it that one of the present head nurses will get her job. Well, each meeting we've had since she resigned has turned out to be just several of the head nurses trying to impress the director with what a fine job they've done—obviously trying to get the assistant's job. We just haven't accomplished what we should have in our meetings during the last month.

Whenever hidden agendas are present in a small group, successful group functioning and decisions are jeopardized. To be successful communicators in small groups, you should avoid personal hidden agendas and should encourage other group members to also avoid such intentions.

DISCUSSION QUESTION

Can you think of a small group in which you were a member and either you or someone else in the group had a hidden agenda? How did the hidden agenda affect the outcome of the group?

Norms

Every small group develops norms. *Norms* are the rules of conduct, standards of participation, and expectations concerning member behavior. Norms evolve and develop within a group, and are explicit or implicit.

Recently, your author was consultant to the Board of Directors of a state funded health care organization. The board (a small group by our definition) was composed of providers (some of whom were nurses) each representing a different health care agency in the community, and consumer/advocates. Many explicit and implicit norms evolved to guide board conduct. Explicit norms were detailed in a ten page single-spaced document and covered items from specific duties of individual board members to parliamentary procedure specifications for conducting board meetings.

In addition, the board developed many implicit norms. One implicit norm was each time the board formed a committee to work on a specific task, the committee would contain at least one provider and at least one consumer/advocate. This norm was implicit—it was not formally written in any document or even openly discussed, however, each member of the board understood the norm, accepted it and acted in accord with it.

However, each subgroup within the board (providers and consumer/advocates) developed their own implicit norms, many of which dealt with overall attitudinal orientation toward the other subgroup. These subgroup implicit norms generally were only understood by the members of the particular subgroup.

Explicit and implicit norms that were understood and accepted by all board members usually were consistent with the overall organizational goals and contributed to successful board functioning. But those implicit norms that were not held by all members generally were contrary to overall organizational goals and adversely affected board functioning.

If you recognize that norms are inherent in a small group, then, to be an effective communicator, you should attempt to contribute in developing group norms that are consistent with group purpose and agreed upon by all members of the group. Generally, the more explicit you can make the norms, the better the overall group functioning.

DISCUSSION QUESTION

In a small group in which you participated, what norms were developed? Did these norms hinder or aid the group? How and why?

Cohesiveness

Associated with every group is a degree of cohesiveness within the group. Cohesiveness means the members' attraction to the group and willingness to band together with other members of the group. Groups can vary from being highly cohesive to having little cohesiveness among members. In general, the more cohesive a group, the more successful the group will be in achieving its goals. However, extreme cohesiveness can lead to groupthink behavior.

In the Board of Directors example used when discussing norms, providers and consumer/advocates were very cohesive within their own subgroup. However, this cohesiveness became so great that groupthink phenomena developed that hindered overall board functioning. Once the implicit subgroup norms were verbally expressed to the entire group (through a technique to be described later) certain inaccurate perceptions were revealed. When these perceptions were accurately clarified and modified, the extreme cohesiveness of the subgroups became less but the overall cohesiveness of the board increased and the board was able to function more effectively.

When in a small group, you should recognize that group cohesiveness is usually very beneficial in fostering effective communication, and you should attempt to nurture cohesiveness whenever possible. But be careful of extreme cohesiveness especially in subgroups of a larger group.

DISCUSSION QUESTION

What degree of cohesiveness was present in a group in which you participated? How did this level of cohesiveness affect the group and group goals? Why?

Techniques for More Effective Small Groups

Many communicative techniques have been developed to help groups function more efficiently and effectively. These techniques have met with varying degrees of success in varying situations. While not detailing all of these techniques and their relative merits, we will discuss two techniques, brainstorming and Nominal Group Technique (NGT) that can, in many circumstances, be used in nursing small groups to improve the group's functioning.

Brainstorming. Brainstorming is a technique in which all members of a group are encouraged to express their ideas concerning a topic. Any idea is acceptable for a brainstorming session. In fact, the wilder the idea the better. As large a *quantity* of ideas as possible is desired. During brainstorming sessions all criticism of others' ideas is withheld, and attempts are made to combine and improve on ideas already expressed. It is usually helpful in brainstorming sessions to have one group member record ideas on a chalkboard or in a similar manner so that all members of the group can visually see and refer to ideas that have been expressed.

When can you, in a small group setting, use brainstorming? Brainstorming can be applied at any time during a small group discussion. It is appropriate when there appears to be no clear-cut course of action or solution to a particular plan or problem. It is also appropriate when members of the group come from different backgrounds and/or are not familiar with each other.

What can you expect from the use of brainstorming? Brainstorming allows group members to "see where others are coming from" on a particular issue, and helps spawn new ideas from members.

What are the limitations of brainstorming? As beneficial as brainstorming can be, it is not always appropriate. If the plan or problem under discussion is too broad, the group is unlikely to obtain sufficient relevant ideas to be of use. Brainstorming should only be attempted when time is not severely restricted—brainstorming takes time and cannot be rushed if it is to be effective. In addition, brainstorming will only work if all group members are willing and able to withhold criticism of others' ideas during the brainstorming session.

We recently observed good use of brainstorming by a small group of nurses. The nurses were involved in planning a day camp program for approximately sixty physically handicapped children. Camp was to be held on the grounds of a local rehabilitation center in midsummer. Outside temperature could be expected to be in excess of 90°F. The nurses' specific task was how to prevent sun and heat-related distress to the children. Most of the planned activities were scheduled for out-of-doors; there were few areas of shade on the center's grounds.

During the brainstorming session, the nurses made scores of statements concerning potential solutions. A few of these statements are presented below to show you the type of statements made in successful brainstorming, the evolution of ideas during brainstorming, and the type of product resulting from successful brainstorming.

"It's too bad we don't have an air conditioned gym ... Or at least a bunch of 40-foot shade trees ... What about making sure each child is taken inside the center for at least 10 minutes out of every hour ... How about umbrellas for each child ... It would be nice if we had a circus tent ... A tent, that's a great idea, but where would we get one ... I could get tents from the Boy Scouts, but they would be very small ... Hey, there's an Army Reserve Medical Unit in town, they might have a large tent we could use."

As a result of this brainstorming session, the Army Reserve was contacted and they were able to supply a large field hospital tent that was set up on the center's grounds. The tent provided the necessary shade and the camp was conducted without any serious heat related problems experienced by the children.

Nominal Group Technique (NGT). While brainstorming can be used in a wide variety of nursing situations, it may not be appropriate when clearly defined problems or issues are of a major importance and group members have strong vested interests. For such major defined issues and problems, a technique that can often be used very successfully was developed by Andre Delbecq and Andrew Van de Ven in 1968, described by Delbecq, Van de Ven, and David Gustafson (1975), that is called Nominal Group Technique, or simply NGT.

NGT involves having all members of a group generate ideas as in brainstorming but, unlike brainstorming, ideas are generated by each group member working *silently,* but in each other's presence, and recorded on a sheet of paper by the individual generating the ideas. After working silently for about five to ten minutes, each individual in the group is asked in round-robin fashion to present one item from the prepared list. These items are recorded for all to see on a flipchart or chalkboard but no indication is recorded concerning who generated the item.

After all group members have contributed an item, the process starts over again until all ideas that members wish to contribute have been posted. No discussion is allowed during this portion of NGT. After all items have been posted, any member of the group is allowed to ask for clarification, but *not evaluation,* of any item on the list.

Once items are clarified, each member of the group is given a sheet of paper and asked to rank order the five or so items most preferred. It is easiest to have people use a system of ranking in which the most preferred item is given the highest possible value. For example, if each person lists five most preferred items, the most preferred could be given a value of 5, the second most preferred a value of 4 and so on. These rankings are then collected anonymously, the ranks summed for each item and a score obtained for each item. The items receiving the highest score should then be discussed in open session in which all group members are encouraged to analyze, criticize, and even express disagreements concerning these items.

If agreement can be reached on a single plan, solution, etc., the NGT process ceases and has been successful. If agreement cannot be reached, the group members are asked to revote (rerank) the items and the process repeats from that point. This reevaluation process can be repeated as many times as necessary.

A slightly modified version of NGT was used by your author as consultant for the Board of Directors mentioned in our discussion of norms and cohesiveness. The NGT session lasted approximately three hours and was conducted to solve a major, specific problem: to identify precisely the function of this Board of Directors.

The consultant began the meeting by asking each board member to take out a sheet of paper and to write answers to three questions: (1) What are the major goals of the overall organization? (2) What are the major goals of the Board of Directors? (3) What are your personal major goals in the organization and as a member of the board?

Members were instructed not to identify themselves in their answers. All responses were to be anonymous. After board members completed writing their answers, the consultant collected the response sheets. On a chalkboard placed so that all could see, the consultant wrote randomly selected responses to the first question. No discussion was allowed during this process. After all responses were recorded, it was clear there was unanimous agreement on the overall goal of the organization—the essence of each answer was the same.

The process was repeated for the second question concerning the board's goal. However, when all responses were recorded, no unanimous answer was evident. Board members were asked to rank the responses in terms of agreement, and discussion was held concerning the rankings. This process was repeated several times until two "answers" emerged, each with equal support. The providers unanimously agreed to one answer; the consumer/advocates to the other.

In discussion that followed, the implicit norms of each subgroup were revealed as was evidence of groupthink phenomena and inaccurate perceptions. The consultant's major task during this time was to ensure that the participants only spoke in terms of reports and withheld personal criticisms of other board members. This process was stressful for all involved. However, once perceptions had been accurately clarified and modified, *all* board members were able to agree on a single answer to the question of the board's goal.

Many other issues were discussed during the NGT session. By what has been described, we hope you have gained some insight into NGT and how you might use NGT in nursing small groups.

There is no guarantee for success when using NGT. This fact, plus the time and effort demands placed on group members using NGT and the potential for heated discussion by group members, makes NGT appropriate only for *major* issues or problems of which resolution is so critical as to warrant the demands and risks of NGT.

SUMMARY

We began this chapter by presenting considerations relating to your involvement in interviews with other health care team members. In such interviews, if patient health care issues are involved, your primary responsibility is to ensure patient welfare. When interacting with health care colleagues, you need to assume the role of interviewer and be Rhetorically Sensitive just as when interacting with patients.

In an interview situation with another nurse, both of you can often assume the role of interviewer. However, in situations such as appraisals or reprimands, one nurse must be the interviewer, the other the interviewee. You should conduct appraisals and reprimands in a direct face-to-face manner; limit statements to reports, if at all possible; use threats only as a last resort and only if you are able to carry them out; and avoid any demonstration of anger. If you are an interviewee, you should plan and prepare for the interview just as if you were the interviewer even though focus is on preparation of answers not questions.

When communicating with a physician, you should recognize that you are a cooperative partner in providing health care. You should follow a physician's orders concerning medication and medical procedures but do not hesitate to question these orders if you have sufficient evidence or concerns that a patient's welfare could be at stake. It is advocated that you be assertive but not aggressive when communicating with physicians by accepting and enacting the role and responsibilities of interviewer.

When interacting with non-nurse, non-physician health care team members, we have reiterated principles presented earlier and have emphasized your need to clarify role relationships and clarify terminology used.

We have discussed you as member of numerous small groups—a small group being defined as 3 to 12 people mutually interacting to achieve some overall goal. We presented characteristics of effective leaders and ways of organizing and leading group discussion. Several group phenomena such as groupthink, hidden agendas, norms and cohesiveness were discussed. Finally, we described brainstorming and Nominal Group Technique, two techniques you can use to help groups function more efficiently and effectively.

The last chapter shall expand on what has been presented to help you more successfully communicate in large organizational settings and in one-to-many public speaking situations.

References

Brilhart, J. K. *Effective group discussion* (3rd ed.). Dubuque, Iowa: Wm. C. Brown Company Publishers, 1978, pp. 37-42, 140, 163-166, 190-192, 220-222.

Delbecq, A. L., Van de Ven, A. H., & Gustafson, D. H. *Group techniques for program planning: A guide to nominal group and delphi processes.* Glenview, IL: Scott, Foresman and Company, 1975, pp. 7-10, 40-82.

Janis, I. L. *Victims of groupthink.* Boston: Houghton Mifflin Company, 1973.

Suggested Readings

Small Group Communication

Applbaum, R. L. *Group discussion* (2nd ed.). Modules in Speech Communication. Palo Alto, California: Science Research Associates, Inc., 1981.
A condensed overview of problem solving and informational sharing in groups. Emphasis is placed on group discussion development and implementation.

Brilhart, J. K. *Effective group discussion* (4th ed.). Dubuque, Iowa: Wm. C. Brown Company Publishers, 1982.
A comprehensive text on small group communication and group discussion techniques. Thorough treatment of small group variables and processes. Based throughout on sound research findings.

CHAPTER 5

Communicating in Health Care Organizations and Public Speaking

Nursing interviews and small group communication almost always take place within a larger context—the context of formal organization such as a hospital, an educational institution, a federal, state, or local governmental agency, or a national or local health care agency. If you hope to be a successful communicator, you cannot ignore the influence of these organizations on you and people with whom you interact.

In the first part of this chapter we shall discuss communicating within health care organizations. Focus will be placed on understanding the nature of large organizations and communication processes at work in such organizations.

The second portion of the chapter will be devoted to you as communicator in a different context—situations in which you must speak to large groups of people. In our presentation concerning public speaking, emphasis will be placed on some specific practical guidelines and techniques you can employ in preparing and giving a public speech.

NURSING AND ORGANIZATIONAL COMMUNICATION

Whenever more than 12 people interact to attain a common goal, we shall define the communicative configuration as an organization. The distinction between "organization" and "small group" is somewhat arbitrary (more than 12 individuals versus 3 to 12), however, there are reasons for the distinction.

Observation and research indicate that as more people are added to a group, certain phenomena occur and certain relational considerations develop that were not present when smaller numbers of people were involved. Some of these organizational factors are linked to issues of control and coordination within the group. If more than 12 people are involved, it is very difficult for any one individual to control and coordinate all group activities—these functions must somehow be "shared" by more than one member of the group.

Our concern in this chapter is you as a member of *large* health care organizations. In such large organizations, not only do issues of control and coordination become important but many other organizational issues influence your ability to function and to communicate.

An Overview of Nursing Organizational Considerations

Within any organization in which you work, countless organizational factors are present that have direct impact on you. Issues such as leadership, motivation, decision making and problem solving procedures and practices, local, state, and national laws, and financial and political restrictions all affect you in your day-to-day interactions.

In addition, daily organizational communicative procedures, practices, and events directly influence your ability to successfully communicate.

We could write countless pages and still not be able to identify all the organizational factors and influences relating to your life as nurse communicator in any large health care organization. But rather than attempt such a task, we have picked a few comments made by our nurse respondents in the hope that they will impress upon you the multitude and variety of organizational concerns. The question was asked of our nurse respondents, "In large health care organizations, what are the main communication problems you have?" Five representative answers received were as follows:

(1) In our hospital we have eight nursing units. One of the biggest problems we have is getting information filtered down to everyone in these units. We do work seven days a week, 24 hours a day. We have people that are off on vacations and holiday times, on days off. We have head nurse meetings twice a month, things are discussed with the head nurses; the head nurses are supposed to go back and have unit meetings with all of their people. Now this is where the problem is because if they have a unit meeting and they have people off; the difficulty is getting the information to these people that are off. A head nurse cannot have a unit meeting and

have all of her people from three shifts there. It is almost impossible. So we do use communication books. They write notes in that. They keep minutes of their unit meeting and they are posted so everybody can read them but reading minutes is not always the same as orally discussing with people.

(2) My main problem in a large hospital like I'm working in now is just to figure out who does what and who has what. Like just yesterday, I needed a special baby formula. I called Central Service because they're the one's who stock our shelves. They said, no, we don't have it, Dietary has it. Dietary said, no, we don't have it, Central Supply has it. Okay, I called Central Supply and they said, no, Pharmacy has it. It was insane. I mean I spent twenty minutes on the phone for a bottle of baby formula that should have been on the shelf. There are just too many people that could have what you need.

(3) In my particular agency we have people and groups all over the state. The people in charge of the overall organization seem to be very good at sending out directives but they don't seem to be able to listen to the concerns and problems of the people in the field.

(4) The biggest problem I see is consistency of information. I may get a memo from the hospital administration stating something is going to occur or something like that. A physician may tell me something different. Another nurse may have yet another story. Any one of them or none of them could be correct.

(5) Considering the fast pace that we are often subjected to and the number of people that we work with, we often don't fully understand all of the organizational factors involved in situations and I think this lack of knowledge in many situations tends to cause problems or make an existing problem worse. As an example, on each floor, we have Standard Operating Procedure (SOP) manuals that describe the way certain procedures should be done. Many times a nurse or an aide will be told to do a procedure, even something as simple as taking particular vital signs, and they'll question why it needs to be done. The response they often get is: "Well, that's what you're supposed to be doing. It's SOP." If people would just bother to check the manuals, often times there is a very good rationale for doing something in a particular way. But then again, there are situations that just don't fit the rationale of the SOP. It's a real problem—you need some continuity in the hospital, but then again you get situations that just aren't standard.

These examples, we hope, impress upon you the variety of organizational communication concerns and problems that you may experience. Also, you should recognize that many of these organizational and organizational communication problems cannot be solved by you, the individual nurse.

Does this mean that you cannot have any effect upon the quality of organizational communication and the overall organization?

By no means. *The more effective individual nurses are in their individual day-to-day communicative interactions, the more effective the overall health care organization.* We will attempt to explain this statement by examining the nature of health care organizations.

The Nature of Health Care Organizations

Large health care organizations are like any large human organization in that they are composed of many individuals in many groups and subgroups joined together for some common goal or purpose. Individuals and groups make up every organization, but every organization is more than simply these individuals and groups.

An organization is an entity unto itself which has certain characteristics. In 1972, W. Charles Redding, a leading authority on organizational communication, listed nine characteristics of human organizations. These characteristics are summarized in Figure 12. Let's examine a few key aspects of these characteristics as they relate to you as communicator in large health care organizations.

Organizational members occupy role positions and organizations require division of labor. Every member of every organization has a specified role within that organization. This book is intended for nurses directly involved in primary patient care. Such nurses have specified roles within a health care organization and are expected to behave in accord with these roles which involve *patient care* not managing the organization.

Thus, if you are a member of our intended audience, your organizational role does not generally involve directly facilitating organizational communication. However, you exercise the ultimate power over the

FIGURE 12 *Universal Characteristics of Human Organizations*

An organization is characterized by:
1. Members occupying role positions, in which they are expected to behave, and communicate, in ways appropriate for these roles.
2. Division of labor, which implies varying degrees of job specialization.
3. Status hierarchy consisting of "superiors" and "subordinates" which exists for coordination and control.
4. A communication network, or more accurately, a network of networks.
5. Combination of groups.
6. Combinations of coalitions, factions, or alliances.
7. Being a process which is dynamic and constantly in flux—always changing.
8. Interdependence, or interlocking, of activities.
9. Systems for processing inputs to produce outputs.

organization, for your effectiveness directly influences the effectiveness of the organization.

Nurses in organizational roles of high administrative duties should refer to W. Charles Redding's book, *The Corporate Manager's Guide to Better Communication,* in the PROCOM series, for specific guidelines on managing organizational communication.

In all organizations, for the organization to be effective, tasks must be divided among members—members become specialists in particular areas.

In organizations involving health care delivery, it is important to have physicians, nurses, technicians, etc., with each group having distinct responsibilities and capabilities. It is also important for each of these groups to have members who become experts in particular areas— no one nurse, for example, can know all there is to know about the many different types or aspects of nursing.

Each of you as a nurse working in some health care organization is a specialist to some degree in some specific area. Also, the larger the organization in which you work, the more specialization that is required in the organization, and the more that develops within the organization.

In terms of being effective organizational communicators, you, the nurse, need *not* be all things to all people, but rather recognize that in a large health care organization, you have your specialty and your expertise and others have their specialties and expertise. For the organization to function effectively, members must communicate in such a manner as to share and aid one another, *not* compete with one another.

DISCUSSION QUESTION

What is your particular organizational role? How does that role relate to the roles of others in the organization? What can you "supply" these other people? What can they "supply" you?

Organizations must have status hierarchy. As we mentioned, key issues in organizations are coordination and control. To coordinate and control an organization there must be superior/subordinate (i.e., status) relationships. Organizations would not be organizations if all members worked individually. In order for individuals to work collectively in an organization, it requires that control and coordination be supplied through status relationships.

A common mistake made in organizations, including health care organizations, is to assume that communication responsibility is the same as organizational control, from the top down, from the supervisor to the subordinate. We have tried to stress throughout that to be an effective communicator, you must assume communicative responsibility not only with patients and nursing subordinates but also with nursing superiors, physicians, and other health care team members. Effective health care organizational communication means that communication and communication responsibility must be from the top down, and from the bottom up, and laterally across the organization.

Organizations contain communication networks and are combinations of groups, coalitions, factions, and alliances. In every organization, messages must be sent between and among organizational members and groups so that decisions can be made and/or actions taken.

The channels and means by which these messages are sent are referred to as communication networks. These networks range from very formal networks, such as those that follow the "organizational chart," to very informal networks, such as the so-called "grapevine." Groups involved in these networks can also be formal, such as the divisions of a hospital or agency, or informal, such as coalitions, factions, and alliances formed on the basis of individual interests, likes, desires, and needs.

Groups within a health care organization exist for a variety of reasons such as patient care, organizational functioning, and personal concerns of organizational members to name but a few. The different networks serve these diverse objectives to varying degrees.

Generally, formal individual and group concerns in an organization should be communicated through the formal networks, and informal concerns through the informal networks. While this is often the case, it is not necessarily the way organizations function or the way they should function.

To be an effective nurse communicator, you should recognize that a multitude of groups and communication networks among these groups exist in any health care organization. Not only must you recognize this fact, but you must employ these groups and networks in such a manner as to achieve your overall goals—providing effective health care superseding all other goals.

What specifically do these statements mean to you as a nurse? You should identify the formal and informal groups and communication networks in your organization, and communicate by using the "proper" networks between and within the "proper" groups as specified within the organization. *However,* if patient/client welfare is at stake, and the use of the proper networks and/or groups results in unsatisfactory outcomes, do not hesitate to employ alternative communicative methods.

Does this mean, for example, that we recommend that you violate the chain of command? Yes, if that is the only way you can ensure patient/client well-being. Our recommendations concerning use of organizational communication networks are consistent with our recommendations in interviews—follow the generally accepted rules and procedures, however, if you are convinced patient/client welfare is jeopardized by such actions, you can, and must, take the personal risk in violating these rules and procedures.

DISCUSSION QUESTION

In the organization in which you work (or have worked) what are the major formal and informal groups to which you belong? How does information flow within and between these groups and other groups in the organization? Can you think of any instances when the "proper" organizational information flow procedures had to be violated to ensure patient/client welfare?

An organization is a dynamic and interdependent system for processing inputs to produce outputs. All organizations are systems. This is to say that all organizations are made up of individuals and groups, but the system (that is the whole, the organization) is more than simply the sum of these parts. The organization is the parts but it is also something unique by itself.

Organizations as systems are dynamic, not static. To be dynamic is to be constantly changing. This change must be in the direction of growth if the organization is to be successful. If growth does not occur, decay must evolve—organizations cannot remain static.

In addition, to state an organization is a system means that all the components within the organization are linked together and interact with each other. If any single component is changed, *all* other components will be affected in some way.

There is one more aspect of viewing an organization as a system that is particularly important. All systems function by taking some type of input and processing this input to produce an output. In health care organizations, medical and nursing knowledge and skills are brought together and applied to patients/clients, resulting, if the process is successful, in improved health for patients/clients.

Inputs, processes, and outputs in health care organizations are very often in the form of *information*. Information is created and shared through effective communication. Thus, a measure of the effectiveness of an organization as a system is often a measure of the effectiveness of communication within that organization.

These are just a few highlights of what it means when we say a health care organization is a system. Let's attempt to apply these concepts to an organizational communication incident described by one of our nurse respondents:

Last week we had an incident that is still causing a furor. A night nurse in our general medical-surgical ward had a very busy night and overlooked cancelling the diet order for a patient scheduled for surgery at 9 AM. Also, no NPO (nothing by mouth) sign was placed on the patient's bed as is our standard operating procedure.

In the morning, a regular diet tray was sent by the diet kitchen to the ward and an aide gave the patient the tray and the patient proceeded to have breakfast. Our aides don't sit in on morning report and this aide was just returning after her two day break. So she wasn't familiar with the patient.

Surgery had to be cancelled and rescheduled for the following day. The following day's schedule was already full and this meant rearranging the last half of the schedule by moving the minor cases which required less recovery time to the afternoon. Our surgery schedule was extended one hour into an "overtime" period which meant the OR staff had to be paid overtime. We're already on a very tight budget.

There were a couple physicians who were just furious over the whole incident and they filed a formal complaint with the hospital administrator. The administrator called in the chief nurse, and . . .

In this example, we see where apparent isolated communicative actions of a single nurse had effects throughout an entire health care organization. If the information input available to the night nurse had been transmitted and processed by the aide, an output could have been attained in which surgery was performed at the scheduled time. However, the "correct" input was not transmitted, the aide enacted the wrong process and an unsatisfactory output (surgery being cancelled) resulted. This output affected not only the individuals directly involved in the situation, but individuals and groups throughout the organization.

This example also demonstrates the dynamic nature of an organization. Because of the incident, the organization has been changed, if in no other respect than relationships between organizational members have been strained. If nothing is done to lessen this stress, the ability of the organization to function properly will be adversely affected—in other words, the organization will decay.

If decay is to be prevented and growth promoted, what can be done? One action that should be taken is development of communicative procedures to help prevent an incident like this occurring again. One such procedure might be to have the aides, especially those returning from their breaks, listen to shift change reports. Can you think of other actions that would help this organization grow?

This example shows the dynamic and interdependent system aspects involved in the processing of information within a health care organization. As a nurse in a health care organization, it is important to consider the systems effects of your communicative actions.

DISCUSSION QUESTION

Can you think of an apparent isolated communication incident in a health care organization in which you work (or have worked) that had impact throughout the organization? If so, analyze the incident in terms of the system's concepts we have presented.

In this brief look at organizations, we have only discussed a very few aspects of organizational communication. The one point to be emphasized for nurses directly involved in primary nursing care: The more successful communicator you are in your day-to-day interactions with individuals (patients, other nurses, physicians, and other health care team members), the more likely the health care organization is to be successful.

THE NURSE AS PUBLIC COMMUNICATOR

At times you will have to communicate in a one-to-many setting or, as it is most often called, a public speaking situation. For many nurses (and for many people in general) public speaking can be a very anxiety producing and stressful event, but it doesn't have to be a negative experience.

Few of our nurse respondents reported anticipating when they began their nursing careers that they would have to give public speeches. However, almost all of our respondents stated that during their nursing careers, they have, in fact, had to give public speeches.

The type of actual public speaking situations described by our respondents included: nursing in-services concerning nursing procedures or nursing organizational issues to groups of nursing aides, technicians, and other nurses; speeches informing other health care professionals or the general public about services provided by a particular group of nurses or health care agency; speeches to lay people about health related issues such as breast cancer self-examinations, CPR training, childhood immunization programs, and childbirth or parenting preparation; speeches to the general public, health care professionals, or governmental groups urging adoption of particular legislative action; and speeches at professional meetings concerning nursing research projects.

How did our respondents view their experiences in nursing public speaking? The responses we received had a wide range from being positive to negative:

I felt it was a great experience, very rewarding. I felt I really accomplished something. I got needed information across to the audience and I felt I corrected some of the misconceptions that the audience had about nurses and nursing.

I have a problem talking to groups. If I sit down, I can talk to anybody individually or small groups—say, less than ten. But when I have to get in front of a large group, I have a hard time. I'm very nervous and I just don't seem to be able to get my ideas across. I'll be truthful, I try to stay away from large group situations whenever I can, but sometimes in my job, I've just got to do it.

DISCUSSION QUESTION

Have you had to give a public speech involving nursing? What were your perceptions of the experience?

Before presenting specific guidelines, it is known that nervousness when giving a public speech is natural, and, in moderate degrees, even desirable. In a public speech, it is your responsibility to affect as many members of the audience as possible, and to accomplish this takes a lot of effort and energy—perhaps more so than any other form of communication. Nervous energy, in moderate degree, can be harnessed and can provide the something extra needed to be an effective public speaker.

The master keys to controlling nervousness and to giving a successful public speech are the same as they are to being an effective interviewer. Those keys are *preparation* and *adaptation*.

Types and Ways of Public Speaking

The first step in public speech preparation is to ask what is the general purpose of the speech, that is, what type of speech is required. Many different schemes have been developed over the years to classify speeches, but the majority of public speeches can be viewed as one of three types: informative, persuasive, or entertaining.

Informative speeches are ones in which facts, opinions, policies, and/or procedures are communicated for the purpose of audience awareness or understanding. Persuasive speeches are ones in which the speaker first informs the audience concerning some issue and then attempts to get the audience to take some specified action with regard to the issue. Entertainment speeches are those in which the speaker simply desires to amuse or entertain the audience.

Few, if any, nurses will have occasion to give a speech to entertain, so we will not discuss this specialized type of speaking, but will restrict ourselves to informative and persuasive speeches—speeches which directly relate to the role of the nurse.

In informative or persuasive speeches, there are four basic ways in which the speech can be presented: impromptu, reading, memorization, and extemporaneous.

Impromptu speeches are speeches given with no preparation; the speaker simply begins speaking "off the top of her or his head." Although there may be some circumstances such as being asked, with no prior warning, during a nursing staff meeting to tell the group about a problem or procedure, potential speaking situations can often be anticipated. If you are able to foresee such situations, you can prepare in advance and avoid having to be completely impromptu.

Reading a manuscript is a specialized art: an art that to be effective requires a great deal of skill and practice. Reading a speech may be appropriate for you whenever subject matter is highly technical and precise, or if wording must be exact either for legal or political reasons. For example, a nurse, as a speaker at a nursing convention, may have to describe a controversial nursing research project. Reading in this case would be very appropriate. However, for most of our intended audience —nurses involved in primary patient/client care—the necessity for ever having to read such a speech is remote.

Memorizing a speech is the most common way inexperienced speakers give a public speech. In our opinion, memorization of a speech is *never* appropriate for you as a nurse. Speech memorization creates a detachment between speaker and audience that is counter to the whole notion of communication and constant adaptive behavior. In addition, if you memorize a speech and forget or mispronounce one word, what happens? The speech is likely to fail. Has this ever happened to you?

The way that we recommend for giving most nursing speeches is called the extemporaneous method. Extemporaneous means the speech is prepared but not written out, not memorized. The remainder of this chapter will be devoted to discussing how to prepare and give an extemporaneous speech.

Outlining an Extemporaneous Speech

There are many effective ways of constructing and outlining an extemporaneous speech. We will present one way to prepare that can be applied to the majority of nursing public speaking situations you are likely to encounter.

The first step in preparing an outline is to conduct a preoutline analysis. The basic principles are the same in analyzing a public speaking situation as were discussed in analyzing an interview situation.

What is the general purpose of the speech—to inform or persuade? What is the specific purpose? The specific issue you are attempting to communicate must be precisely formulated and kept clearly in mind. Who is your audience? Information and language appropriate for one audience may be very inappropriate for another audience. What is your audience's general attitude and prior knowledge concerning the topic of your speech? These issues directly affect how your speech will be perceived and what type response you will elicit by various types of statements.

Once this preoutline information has been determined, you are ready to begin preparing your outline. There are many ways to construct and outline a speech. One method which can be successfully adapted to a great number of nursing public speaking situations is a technique known as Monroe's Motivated Sequence.

Monroe's Motivated Sequence

Over sixty years ago, Alan Monroe, a pioneer in the study of speech communication, detailed a manner to construct a persuasive speech based upon the natural mind process that all of us use whenever we persuade ourselves to do anything.

An assumption made in this description is that before a person can be persuaded, the person must be informed. The persuasive process described by Monroe begins with a description of the informative process.

Monroe's scheme, known as the Motivated Sequence, has been described by Alan Monroe and Douglas Ehninger (1967) as well as in many previous and subsequent versions of Monroe's basic book. It is presented in Figure 13. The first three steps can be used to construct a speech to inform. If the final two steps are added, the informative process is expanded and transformed into the persuasive process. Thus, the total five steps can be used to construct a speech to persuade.

Using the Motivated Sequence

The Motivated Sequence is the skeleton upon which we recommend building informative and persuasive speech outlines. Use the first three steps (Attention, Need, Satisfaction) in informative speeches; use all five steps (Attention, Need, Satisfaction, Visualization, Action) in persuasive speeches.

Since the time Monroe first described the Motivated Sequence,

FIGURE 13 Monroe's Motivated Sequence

Attention
The first step toward persuasion involves gaining and directing our attention to the issue at hand. Unless our attention is focused, we cannot be persuaded.

Need
Once attention is aroused, if we are to be persuaded, we must realize that we have some sort of need or problem that requires resolution.

Satisfaction
After a need or problem is recognized, persuasion requires that we see some manner of satisfying or solving this need or problem. The specifics of the solution must be clear.

Visualization
To recognize something as a solution to a need or problem is not by itself sufficient to persuade us to take any concrete steps to enact the solution. We must somehow visualize ourselves (that is, picture ourselves) personally enjoying the benefits of the solution.

Action
Having pictured ourselves actually implementing the solution, all that is required for persuasion to occur is a statement of definitive action.

---

public speaking experts have developed many sophisticated techniques to actually implement the Motivated Sequence but the basic sequence has remained unchanged. While we cannot describe all of these techniques, we can present a basic procedure that you can employ.

We provide an actual speech outline and transcript in Figures 14 and 15 to demonstrate use of the Motivated Sequence. The speech evolved in the following situation: A local health care community agency has been requested to prepare and conduct a series of parenting classes for parents of children enrolled in a local Head Start preschool program. Classes will be presented by nurses and child development experts. The director of the Head Start program has informed the parents that the classes will be offered and the times at which they will be offered. However, he is concerned that the parents do not understand the benefits to be gained from the classes, and that many parents will not attend. He has requested the agency send a nurse to talk to the parents at an opening orientation meeting of the program. His desire is that the nurse can show the parents the relevance of the classes and persuade them to attend the classes. An audience of between 40 and 50 parents is anticipated. The audience will be predominantly mothers, but a few fathers can be anticipated.

Read and study this outline and speech carefully. You will note on the outline only key words and phrases were written. Important preoutline information was actually written on the outline.

FIGURE 14 Example of Nursing Speech Outline

Preoutline Information
General purpose: to persuade.
Specific purpose: to convince parents of children enrolled in a Head Start preschool program of the need for their active participation in parenting classes.
Audience: Approximately 40 to 50 low-income parents—mostly mothers, but a few fathers may be in attendance.
Audience attitude: Probably receptive, but few probably understand the relevance or actual content of the parenting classes.

Outline
I. *Attention Step* — Welcome. Television without picture tube. Analogy to Head Start.
   (personal greeting, analogy using rhetorical questions)
II. *Need Step*
   A. *Statement* — Need to help Head Start help your child. Parents need skills.
   B. *Illustration* (explanation) — Child in Head Start short time. With parent much longer. Work together.
   C. *Ramification*
      (explanation) — Reasons parents place child in Head Start.
      (restatement) — You want to help your child.
      (detailed example) — Conversation with woman. Prepared for childbirth, not prepared for parenting.
      (specific instance) — Learn parenting by doing or what remember from childhood.
      (analogy) — Walk tight rope, but no training.
      (testimony) — Direct quote from Piaget (if seems appropriate). If not — general statement.
   D. *Pointing* — See need. How do we do it?
III. *Satisfaction Step*
   A. *Initial Summary*
      1. Parents' natural frustrations and uncertainties.
      2. Child's progressive development.
      3. Parents' contributions to child's growth.
   B. *Detailed Information*
      1. a. Frustrations.
            3-month-old crying all day.
            2-year-old saying "no" to everything.
            3-year-old crying when babysitter comes.
            4-year-old writing with felt-tip pen on wall.
         b. Uncertainties
            Want to slap child—stop.

	Not solve problem.
	May hurt child.
	Feelings okay, but not okay to lose control.
	2. Developmental stages of child.
	3-month-old—self-centered, get someone to help.
	2-year-old—autonomous, recognize, distract.
	3-year-old—attachment, fine when leave, know babysitter.
	4-year-old—creativity, provide outlet.
	3. Parents' contributions to development.
	a. Structure experiences to aid learning.
	b. React to child's level.
	c. Be firm but don't traumatize (hurt) child.
C. *Final Summary*	1. Natural frustrations and uncertainties.
	2. Progressive development of children.
	3. Contributions parent can make.
IV. *Visualization*	Want children out of hair for a few hours a day? Or, want children to succeed in school and life? If you help—will succeed; if you don't help—probably won't succeed.
V. *Action*	To help child, attend parenting classes. Start next week, this time.
	Questions?

FIGURE 15   Example of Nursing Speech

I. Attention	I would like to welcome you today and thank you for coming. Let me begin by asking you a question. What if you didn't have a television set in your home? And you decided that for your children you were going to go out and buy one. Would you buy a television set without a picture tube? Of course, you wouldn't. You'd want to make sure that you got a set that worked properly and that your children would be able to watch. Well, you have obtained for your children something much more valuable than a television set. And that is, you have gotten for them the opportunity to be in the Head Start program. However, this gift that you have gotten them, just like our television set we were talking about, lacks a main component, the main piece, and without this component it will not operate.
II. Need	
A. Statement	You, as parents, need to help the Head Start program help your child. And you need to have certain skills to do this.
B. Illustration (explanation)	Let's think about this for a moment. Your child is in the Head Start program only for a short time each day. However, the child is with you, the parent, for a much longer time. Only if the Head Start program and the parents work together can your children benefit.

The Nurse as Public Communicator 113

C. Ramification
  (explanation)

  (restatement)

  (detailed example)

Most parents place their children in the Head Start program to get certain things for their children that the parents didn't get themselves as children. The parents recognize that their children need help. And you as parents really do want to help your child. But how are we prepared to do this?

Let me tell you an example of a woman I was talking to just a few days ago. She was telling me about some of her feelings. She said, "You know, when I was expecting my child, there were classes to help me prepare and get through the delivery. They told me what to expect, what to do. The nurses and doctors gave me all kinds of information about childbirth. I was really prepared for childbirth. But you know I just haven't been prepared at all about how to raise a child."

  (specific instance)

For most of us as parents, our preparation for raising children is simply by doing it or what we can remember from our own childhood. We learn by our mistakes—it is trial and error.

  (analogy)

It's like we are asked to walk a tightrope above a deep canyon. But we have no preparation on how to do that. It's like if we get across, okay, but if we don't, it's just too bad.

  (testimony-general)

Many books have been written by psychologists stressing the importance of parent skills and how necessary these parent skills are in helping a child to develop. Without parents doing their jobs, the child is unlikely to develop to do the types of things that child is capable of. So, we see that we as parents need to help our children. But how are we going to do it?

D. Pointing

III. Satisfaction
  A. Initial Summary

What I want to talk about briefly with you today are three major points that you as parents need to recognize and understand.

  The first of these is that parents have natural frustrations and uncertainties. By the very nature of us being parents, there are certain things that our children will do that will concern or upset us. And there will be situations that we just don't know how to handle.

  Another thing I want to talk to you about is that children go through a progressive developmental sequence. By this I mean that children are constantly growing—not just physically but also emotionally and socially.

  The third thing I want to talk to you about is just what you can do to contribute to your child's growth.

  B. Detailed Information

Let's look first at some of these frustrations that we all have.

  You have a 3-month-old at home. And the 3-month-old has been crying all day. The child doesn't have a fever, has been fed, has a clean diaper on—there seems to be no reason why the child should be crying. But the child continues to cry and there's nothing you do that stops the child from crying.

You have a 2-year-old and every time you ask him to do something, he says, "No, no I won't. No."

Or you have a 3-year-old and you're wanting to go out for the evening. But your 3-year-old just starts crying and screaming as soon as the babysitter comes and just won't stop.

Or you have a 4-year-old and your 4-year-old has just taken a felt tip pen and scribbled all over a freshly painted wall in your living room.

We've experienced things like this? Yes, I can see by your reactions that we have. Now we as parents have many frustrations and uncertainties. In the examples I've given, maybe our feelings are we just want to slap the child—we just want to "beat the heck" out of the child. But stop! Don't! It's okay to think about wanting to slap the child in situations like I've described, but we shouldn't because in these type situations slapping will not solve the problem and besides we may hit the child much harder than we intended and we may really hurt the child. What I want to stress to you today is that it's okay to have these feelings, but it's *not* okay to lose control of your feelings.

One thing we have to do is to consider the progressive developmental sequence that children go through. "Progressive developmental sequence"—that's a big term. What does it mean?

Like the 3-month-old that we were talking about. The 3-month-old is very, very self-centered. All that child knows is about himself. The whole world is himself and he really has no knowledge about your feelings. Crying is his way of telling you that something is wrong. The child is saying, "I'm not comfortable." Maybe you've been uptight all day—the car wouldn't start, you spilled a gallon of milk all over the floor, you've got a headache. Babies do sense when you're not relaxed. Maybe what you could do is have a grandmother come over and take care of the child for an hour or so. Give yourself a chance to relax, and if you do, maybe you'll find your child will relax too.

What about the 2-year-old? The 2-year-old is likely in the stage where he is very autonomous. By this I mean, he wants to do everything by himself—he wants to show that he is really a person. What can you, the parent, do? The first thing you can do is simply recognize this. The child is not being cruel to you, he is just showing, in his own way, that he is a person. You as the parent, however, have to make it clear to him that you mean what you say. You can do this at times by just the tone of your voice. Another thing that can often help is to distract the child's attention to something else. You may want to pick up the child and take him to another room—show him something different. Anything to focus his attention on something different.

What about your 3-year-old? What is the 3-year-old doing by crying as soon as the babysitter comes? The 3-year-old is at a stage when she is feeling a strong attachment to you—she doesn't want to let go of you. She's trying everything she can to hold onto you. What you'll find usually is that if you just leave and go out and leave the child with the babysitter, within a couple of minutes after you're out the door, the child will stop crying. It's important though that the child knows the babysitter. If you're getting a new sitter, you could ask the sitter to come over a day or so before you need her and just visit with you and the child. Let the sitter and child get to know each other.

What about the 4-year-old who just scribbled on your wall? He sees the wall as a nice place to express his creativity. Four-year-olds are often in a stage when they want to be creative—they want to do new things. When he does something like mark-up the wall, you have to stop and ask yourself, "What have I provided for him so that he can express his ideas?" Is there a chalkboard or large piece of cardboard or anything that he can use to mark on? Give him soap crayons, big pieces of paper, things like this. Let him express his creativity, but give him the chance to do this in a way acceptable to you.

Now, what can we as parents do to contribute to the development of our child? We can do several things.

First, we have to build the experiences for the child to aid in his learning. In other words, we have to work at providing the right environment for the particular child. We have to provide the child with things that the child needs at the child's particular stage of development.

Second, we need to react to the child at the child's level of knowledge, thinking, feeling, and his ability to get along with other people. Each child at each age is different—we need to know where our particular child is at in terms of his particular development.

And finally, we must be very certain that we, as parents, are firm and consistent in our expressions of what the child is allowed to do and what the child is not allowed to do. We must be firm in letting the child know

	we are in charge. But being firm does *not* mean that we physically or emotionally hurt, or as it is called "traumatize," the child.
C. Final Summary	These are things we have to do if we want to help our child. We have to recognize that we, as parents, have natural frustrations and uncertainties. We have to recognize that the child goes through a progressive development. And we have to personally contribute to the child's growth.
IV. Visualization	What do we want for our children? Do we want our children just out of the way for a few hours a day? So we put them in Head Start to "get them out of our hair." Or do we want the child to really succeed in school and in life? I think by just being here today, you're telling me you want them to succeed. With your help they can succeed, without your help, they probably won't.
V. Action	To help you help your child, I want you to attend the parenting classes which you've already heard about and which will be held each week at this time, starting next week. In these classes you'll be able to discuss your concerns, frustrations, and problems about your own children; you'll get a deeper understanding of your children; and you'll gain confidence in your abilities as parents. Please come to the classes for your children's sake.
	If you have any questions, at this time, I'll be happy to answer them.

The Attention Step. In the sample speech, a personal greeting and an analogy using rhetorical questions (questions which prompt the audience to seek an answer in their own minds) were used to gain and direct attention. There are countless ways of successfully gaining attention. Personal greetings, use of analogy, and rhetorical questions are but a few possible ways to gain attention.

The important point to remember in gaining attention is that your audience's interest must be gained *and* directed to the rest of the speech. A common mistake in public speaking is to think of an interesting attention device but one that does not relate to the rest of the speech. In such a case, the attention step *and* the overall speech are likely to be ineffective.

The Need Step. In the sample speech, the need step was broken into four substeps—the Statement, Illustration, Ramification, and Pointing.

The Statement was a clear and concise definition of the need or problem that exists for the audience. "You, as parents, need to help the Head Start program help your child. And you need to have certain skills to do this."

The Illustration and Ramification contain supporting materials for the Statement. Supporting materials will be defined as materials which provide explanation and proof of the problem or need upon which the audience's belief and understanding will rest. The seven most commonly used verbal supporting materials are listed in Figure 16. You will note that six of these seven were prepared for use in our sample speech.

The only difference between the Illustration and Ramification steps is that the Illustration contains the one item of supporting material that is considered by the speaker to be the most important; the Ramification contains all of the other supporting materials. In the sample speech, the explanation concerning the amount of time the child spends with the parent was judged by the speaker to be the most important supporting material in the speech. Therefore it was placed in the Illustration step.

There are many reasons for organizing the Need Step in such a manner, not the least of which is that audience reaction or time constraints may dictate that all prepared supporting material may not be used in the actual speech. If a prepared item of support is not used, we want to ensure it is not the most important. In the sample speech, specific quotes from Jean Piaget (a cognitive development expert) were prepared but not used at the end of the Ramification Step.

The number of items of supporting material depends on the specific circumstances involved, such as audience's prior knowledge, time constraints, etc. Use as much support as you judge necessary to ensure that the audience understands the problem. Also, in general, the more variety that can be used in types of support, the greater the chance for a successful speech.

The Pointing Step is simply a brief restatement of the Statement

FIGURE 16 Forms of Verbal Supporting Materials

1. *Explanation*—a simple description of the need or problem
2. *Analogy or comparison*—similarities or differences between something the audience is familiar with and the present need or problem
3. *Detailed example*—an expanded narration of an actual or hypothetical situation in which the need or problem existed
4. *Specific instance*—an undeveloped example involving the need or problem
5. *Statistics*—quantifiable descriptions using numeric symbols
6. *Testimony*—quotes from a generally recognized authority on the subject
7. *Restatement*—saying the same thing in either the same words or different words in order to emphasize

and a lead into the solution. "So, we see that we as parents need to help our children. But how are we going to do it?"

One point must be stressed at this time. From our experience, one of the most common reasons for nurses to be ineffective in public communication is for them to ignore the Need Step. The nurse knows what the problem or need is and assumes the audience also knows. This is a very dangerous assumption for if the audience doesn't realize the specific problem, they are unlikely to understand the importance of the solution.

The Satisfaction Step. The Satisfaction Step is the "heart" of the speech. It is the solution. Many schemes have been developed to organize the Satisfaction Step for specific circumstances. However, the scheme we prefer is the most general and can be applied to almost any public speaking situations the nurse will encounter. The format consists of three parts: the Initial Summary, Detailed Information, and Final Summary. In the Initial Summary, we tell the audience what we are going to do; in the Detailed Information we do it; and in the Final Summary we tell the audience what we have done. Note how the sample speech accomplishes these objectives.

If the speech were to end at this point, we would have an informative speech. If we want to persuade, we need two additional steps.

The Visualization Step. In the Visualization Step we "paint a picture" for the audience. We attempt to help the audience see themselves, even if only momentarily, enjoying the benefits of doing whatever we have described in the Satisfaction Step.

In the sample speech, the speaker attempted to get the audience to imagine what specifically would happen to their children if the parents followed the speaker's advice, or what would happen if they did not follow the advice given in the Satisfaction Step.

The Action Step. If we have been successful to this point in the speech, persuasion will occur if we simply ask the audience to take a specific action in accord with the detailed solution we have presented.

The speaker in our example simply requested that the parents attend the upcoming classes. The more successful the speaker was in this entire process of persuasion, the greater the number of parents who would actually attend the classes.

Speech Content and Delivery

There are two major aspects to any speech: content (what we say), and delivery (how we say it).

It is our position that in nursing public speaking situations, content is most important; delivery is important only insofar as it does not detract from content.

Your job involves communicating information, not putting on a show. As long as you do nothing in delivery to divert attention from the content, you can be a successful public communicator. Examples of delivery factors that draw an audience's attention from content are: "unprofessional" appearance such as inappropriate clothing items and unkempt hair; extreme manifestations of nervousness such as excessive pacing, body swaying, and nervous movement; lack of enthusiasm, failure to maintain eye contact with the entire audience, and instead, staring at the ceiling, floor, or back wall; either repetitive hand gestures or no hand gestures at all; lack of voice vitality because of speech pace too fast or slow, voice pitch forced, or very uneven speaking pace; and lack of speech clarity because of mispronunciations, excessive use of slang or excessive use of fillers such as ah, ah ha, okay, you know, etc.

There are many special techniques that can be employed to ensure delivery is nondetracting, but here we will simply state that your public speaking delivery is effective when it is *natural*. Perhaps the primary key to natural delivery is to keep in mind that you, as a public speaker, are attempting to communicate with each and every member of the audience as an individual.

For those of you who desire in-depth explanation of delivery factors in public speaking (or any other aspect of public speaking), refer to Robert Doolittle's *Professionally Speaking: A Concise Guide* in the PROCOM series.

In addition to analyzing the total situation, preparing an outline, and maintaining a natural delivery, there is one other important issue that you should consider. That issue is practice. Most effective nursing public speeches are rehearsed beforehand. We recommend practicing a speech two or three times *out loud* in someone else's presence.

It is important to hear your own words, and, if possible, have someone reacting nonverbally to those words. If you have no one to be your practice audience, you can speak to a mirror—the important thing is to actually say the words. When you are practicing using an extemporaneous method, you should realize that each time you give the speech, it will be slightly different; the major content will be the same but the details will vary. This variation is desirable for it allows you in the actual speech to adapt to the situation and to the audience.

Also, when you are practicing, if you make a mistake, do not stop, but rather continue and complete the speech. Stopping unconsciously draws your attention to that particular item and, in the actual speech, your unconscious feelings are likely to cause you to have problems at that point in the speech.

One final point concerning practice. Do not practice more than three times. By excessive practicing you tend to memorize and, as previously stated, if the speech is memorized you are unlikely to be an effective public communicator.

Making the Presentation

Having prepared the outline and practiced, you are ready to give the actual speech.

Use natural delivery as we have discussed. Use the outline. Try not to hold onto the outline but have it available to glance at to direct and focus your thoughts. Use visual aids whenever appropriate and possible. Visual aids stress points for your audience, help the audience retain necessary information, and aid you, the speaker, by acting like an outline in helping you direct and focus your thoughts. And above all, keep in mind that effective nursing public speaking like other forms of nursing communication dictates constant adaptive behavior by you.

While not presenting a full description of nursing public speaking, we have attempted to provide a few guidelines that you, the nurse, can incorporate within your professional expertise to be a successful public communicator.

SUMMARY

In this concluding chapter, we expanded our coverage and extended our basic communication concerns and principles to include you as nurse communicator in large health care organizations and in public speaking situations.

We defined an organization as simply more than twelve individuals interacting to attain a common goal. Focus was placed on your involvement in large health care organizations and the multitude of factors that influence your ability to communicate in such organizations. Although you, as a nurse, often have little control over organizational factors, your communicative competence is a major determinant of the effectiveness of the organization.

We examined a few aspects that are particularly salient for you as an organizational nurse communicator such as your role and related communicative responsibilities. These responsibilities are to all organizational components and levels. If patient/client welfare is at stake, you have responsibility to ensure patient/client well-being, even if this means violating organizational rules and procedures.

You must also recognize that every health care organization is a system. This statement has many implications. Your individual communicative actions can, and will, have impact throughout the organization.

The more effective you are in your day-to-day communicative interactions, the more effective the overall health care organization.

At times, you may have to engage in public speaking. Nervousness in such situations is natural. You need to harness this nervousness through preparation and adaptation—the same ingredients needed to be successful in any communicative configuration.

We recommend preparing your informative and persuasive speeches in an extemporaneous manner. This means you prepare an outline, practice, and present—always being willing and able to adapt if necessary.

We recommend using Monroe's Motivated Sequence to form the framework for your speeches. The Motivated Sequence contains five parts. You can construct an informative speech by using the first three of these parts—Attention, Need, and Satisfaction. Simply add the final two parts—Visualization and Action—to form a persuasive speech. An actual outline and speech transcript were provided for you to analyze and use as an example.

In this book, we have presented concerns and principles we believe are essential for successful nursing communication. We have applied these fundamentals to a variety of nursing communicative configurations. By your sharing with us in this process, we hope you have taken important steps in becoming a more successful nurse communicator.

References

Monroe, A. H., & Ehninger, D. *Principles and types of speech communication* (6th ed.). Glenview, IL: Scott, Foresman and Company, 1967, pp. 155-172, 265-287.

Redding, W. C. *Communication within the organization.* New York: Industrial Communication Council, Inc., 1972, pp. 17-21.

Suggested Readings

Organizational Communication

Goldhaber, G. M. *Organizational communication* (3rd ed.). Dubuque, Iowa: Wm. C. Brown Company Publishers, 1983.
An introductory examination of many significant organizational communication variables.

Redding, W. C. *Communication within the organization.* New York: Industrial Communication Council, Inc., 1972.
A comprehensive treatment of organizational communication. Delineates the scope of organizational communication variables and thoroughly summarizes organizational communication research conducted up to 1972. A classic, but one that is very difficult to obtain because of limited printing.

Redding, W. C. *The corporate manager's guide to better communication.* PROCOM Series. Glenview, IL: Scott, Foresman and Company, 1984 (in press).

General Systems Theory

Ruben, B. D., & Kim, J. Y. *General systems theory and human communication.* Rochelle Park, NJ: Hayden Book Company, Inc., 1975.
An advanced and comprehensive examination of General Systems Theory and its relationship to human communication. Contains several major "systems" articles. Requires reader have some understanding of natural and physical sciences and mathematics.

Sutterley, D. C., & Donnelly, G. F. *Perspectives in human development nursing throughout the life cycle.* Philadelphia: J. B. Lippincott Co., 1973.
Detailed application of General Systems Theory principles to the range of nursing activities.

Public Speaking

Doolittle, R. *Professionally speaking: A concise guide.* PROCOM Series. Glenview, IL: Scott, Foresman and Company, 1984 (in press).

Ehninger, D., Gronbeck, B. E., & Monroe, A. H. *Principles of speech communication* (8th brief ed.). Glenview, IL: Scott, Foresman and Company, 1980.
A standard text used for teaching public speaking. Discusses most major aspects involved in public speaking. One of several updated versions of Alan Monroe's classic book in which he first described the Motivated Sequence.

INDEX

Page numbers in italics indicate a figure; page numbers followed by a t indicate a table.

Accenting nonverbal function, 43
Accurate perception, 56, 73
Action step, *110, 112*, 116, 118
Adaptation, 107
Adaptive behavior, 58, 77, 120
Advocate role, 9
Aggressive behavior, 84
Agreement of perception, 56
Aide, and nurse relationship, 78
Alliances, 103
Altman, I., 54
American Association of Critical Care Nurses, 2
The American Nurse, 2
American Nurses Association, 2
ANA, 2
  Resolution of, 2
Analogy
  in attention step, 116
  as verbal support material, *117*
Anger demonstration, 67, 82
  in nursing appraisal, 81
Anxiety, of patient, 64, 68
Appearance, for public speaking events, 119
Appraisals, 80-82, 96
Artifacts, 45t, 49-50
Assertiveness training, 84
Assessment/intervention, 34-35
Attention step, *110, 111, 112*, 116
Attitude
  of audience, *111*
  encoding of, 13
Attitude sets, 13-14
  implications of, 19-21
  Noble Self in, 17-18
  Rhetorical Reflector in, 18
  Rhetorical Sensitivity in, 17
  RHETSEN instrument and, 13, 14t-15t, 20t

Beavin, J., 6
Behavior
  adaptive, 31, 54, 58, 77, 120
  aggressive, 84
  anger and, 81, 82
  assertive, 84
  defensive, 72, 81
  empathetic, 31, 33, 38, 58
  judgmental, 81
  manipulative, 84
  nonverbal, 42-51. *See also* Nonverbal communication
  supportive, 66, 67, 69, 72
Body movement, 44, 45t
  in nonverbal communication, 42, 43
  of public speaker, 119
Brainstorming, 92-93
Brilhart, J. K., 4, 24, 88, 89, 97
Brockreide, W., 26
Burks, D. M., 25

Carlson, R. E., 25
Cash, W. B., 52
Casual-personal distance, 48, 48t
Child
  assessment of, 34, 35
  developmental level of, 67
  and parents of, 66
  touching and, 46
Client, definition of, 9
Closed questions, 36-37, 39t, 41
Clothing, as artifact, 49
Coalitions, 103
Colleagues, interviewing of, 76-86, 96
Combination approach, 72
Combination interview strategy, 33
Communication
  attitude sets in, 13-21
  with child, 66

123

competence in, 12-13
definition of, 4-6, 23
with health care team, 85-86
with infant, 46, 47
inference in, 81
interviewing as, 26-51. *See also*
   Interviewing
leadership and, 89
networks of, 101t, 103
with nonpatient, 76-86, 96
nonverbal, 42-51, 67, 70
for nurses, 7-12
in organizations, 98-106
with patient, 53-75
with physician, 83-85
public speaking as, 106-120, *110, 111, 112-116, 117*
range of, 7
skills of, 3, 4
in small groups, 86-97
training in, 12-13
two-party, 7
Communication in Nursing Practice, 4
Community health nursing, 10
Comparison, as verbal support material, *117*
Complementing nonverbal function, 43
Configurations, 7
Conflict, 57
   in nurse-physician relationship, 83-84
Contradicting nonverbal function, 43
Control, organizational, 102
Coordination, organizational, 102
Co-orientation perspective, 56-58
The Corporate Manager's Guide to Better Communication, 102
Cosmetics, 49
Crable, R. E., 24
Cultural determinants, personal distance as, 49

Darnell, D. K., 24
Decision making, in organizations, 103
Defensive behavior, 70, 81
Delbecq, A., 94, 97
Delivery, of speeches, 118-120
Depression, 57
Detailed example, as verbal support material, *117*
Detailed information in satisfaction step, 118
Direct questions, 36, 39t
Directive interview strategy, 32, 35, 41, 65, 68, 72

Division of labor, within organizations, 101, 101t, 102
Donnelly, G. F., 122
Doolittle, R., 119, 120, 122
Double negative effect, 57

Eadie, W. F., 13, 25
Edwards, B. J., 4, 24
Ehninger, D. E., 109, 121, 122
Emergencies, 33
Empathetic behavior, 31, 33, 38, 58
Encoding, 13
Entertainment speeches, 107
Environmental factors, 45t, 50-51
Explanation, as verbal support material, *117*
Explicit norms, 91
Extemporaneous speeches, 108
   outlining of, 108-109
   practicing of, 119
Eye contact, for public speaker, 119

Face-to-face interaction, appraisals and, 80-82
Fact finding, 33
Factions, 103
Family, 9, 10
Final summary, in satisfaction step, 118
Fingernail polish, 49
Formal network, 103
Fundamentals of interviewing, 52
Funnel sequence, 42

Goldhaber, G. M., 121
Goyer, R., 26
Gronbeck, B. E., 122
Group
   brainstorming in, 92-93
   cohesiveness of, 92
   communication in, 7, 86-97
   discussion in, 89
   dynamics of, 86
   groupthink and, 89-90
   hidden agenda and, 90
   leadership in, 88-89
   log for, *87*
   nominal group technique in, 94-95
   norms of, 91-92
   vs. organization, 98-99
   within organizations, 103
   structure of, 88-89
Groupthink, 89-90
Gustafson, D. H., 94, 97

Index

Hall, E., 48
Hand gestures, of public speaker, 119
Hart, R. P., 13, 25
Hayakawa, S. I., 34
Health care organization,
    communication in, 98-106. See also
    Organization
Health care team, communication with,
    76-86, 96
Hidden agenda, 90
High accuracy, 57
High agreement, 57
Highly scheduled interview, 40
Highly scheduled standardized
    interview, 41
Hospital room, 50
Hospital ward, 11
Hunsberger, M., 5

Ideas, for brainstorming, 93
"Ignorance," 57
Illustration, in need step, 117
Image, of nurse, 1-3
Implicit norms, 91
Impromptu speeches, 108
Infant, nonverbal communication
    and, 46, 47
Inference statement, 34, 35, 81
Informal network, 103
Information, 104
    giving of, 33
    in interviewing, 58-59
    for preoutline, 111
Informative interview, 30
Informative speech, 107, 108
    motivated sequence for, 109-118
Initial summary, in satisfaction step, 118
Interaction, two-party, 26-27
Interdependence, organizational, 104, 105
Interpersonal relationships, 6
    interviewing and, 26-51. See also
    Interviewing
Interpretation, of messages, 6
Interviewee, 29
    nurse as, 82
Interviewing, 26-51
    close of, 58-59, 64, 65
    definition of, 26
    goals of, 30
    inference statements in, 34, 35
    for information, 30
    interviewee role in, 82-83
    judgment statements in, 34, 35

listening in, 27
log for, 28t
misinterpretation in, 81
of nonpatient, 76-86
of patient, 30
    analysis of, 59-61
    configurations for, 63-73
    co-orientation perspective in, 56-58
    monitor observer notes for, 64-73
    observer evaluation of, 62
    patient orientation in, 64-73
    pre-interview evaluation for, 61
of peers, 41t, 80-82
persuasive, 30
pre-interview questioning in, 29t
purpose of, 27, 30-31, 58
questioning in, 36-39
report statement in, 34, 35
responsibilities in, 58-59
schedules for, 40-41
sequencing for, 42
social penetration process in, 54-56, 55t
strategies of, 32-33, 58
    implementation of, 32-42
    statements and, 80-81
of subordinates, 80-82
of superiors, 80-82
for support giving, 30
two-party, 26-27
Intimate personal distance, 48, 48t
Inverted funnel sequence, 42

Jackson, D., 6
Janis, I., 89, 97
Jewelry, 49
Judgmental behavior, 81
Judgmental statement, 34, 35

Kennell, J., 46
Kim, J. Y., 121
Klaus, M., 46
Knapp, M., 43, 44, 52

Language, 85, 86
    for child, 66
    for interview, 42
Leader, 88-89
    vs. leadership, 88
    role of, 12
Leadership, 88-89
    vs. leader, 88

Leading questions, 39, 39t
Licensed practical nurse, 8
Licensure requirements, 2
Listening, in interviewing, 27
Log, for nursing groups, 87

Manipulative behavior, 84
Manuscript reading, 108
"Mechanical" medical service, 3
Media, nurse's image and, 2
Medication, administration of, 30-31
Memorization, of speeches, 108
Message
  communication of, 5
  interpretation of, 6
Meta-perception, 56
Misinterpretation, 81
"Mm-hm," 38, 39t
Moderately scheduled interviews, 40
Monroe, A., 109, 121, 122
Motivated sequence, 109-111, *110, 111, 112-116,* 121
  attention step in, 116
  need step in, 116-117

National League for Nursing, 2
Need sequence, *110, 111, 112, 116*
  support materials for, 117
Nervousness, 107, 119, 121
Networks, 101t, 103
NGT, 94-95
NLN, 2
Noble Self, 17, 18, 22, 79
  implications of, 19
Nominal group technique, 94-95
Nondirect interviewing strategy, 32-33, 35-36, 64, 71, 72
Nonpatient, interviews with, 76-86, 96
Nonscheduled interview, 40
Nonverbal communication, 5, 6, 27, 42-51, 67, 70
  artifacts as, 45t, 49-50
  body motion as, 44
  definition of, 42
  environmental factors as, 45t, 50-51
  functions of, 43-44
  goal attainment and, 44
  paralanguage as, 45t, 48
  personal space as, 45t, 48-49, 48t
  physical characteristics as, 45t, 46
  touching as, 45t, 46
Norms, 91-92

Nurse, and aide relationship, 78
  attitude sets of, 13-21
  behavior of, 31
  and colleague communication, 76-86, 79, 96
  communication needs of, 3, 12-13
  as interviewee, 82-83
  as interviewer, 26-51. *See also* Interviewing
  leadership role of, 12
  licensure requirements of, 2
  and patient relationship, 11, 29
    family in, 9, 10
    personal distance and, 49
  and peers, 29
    communication with, 79, 80-82
    interviews of, 41t
    personal distance and, 49
  and physician relationship, 9, 10
    communication in, 77-78, 83-85, 96
    interview role and, 29
    personal distance and, 49
  professional image of, 1-3, 22-23
    interviewer role and, 79
  as public speaker, 7, 106-120, *110, 111, 112-116, 117*
  roles of, 4, 7-12
    perception of, 7-12
  and subordinate, 29
  and superior, 29

Observer interview evaluation form, 62
Office arrangement, 50
Open questions, 36, 39t
Organization(s), 98-106, 120
  characteristics of, 101-106, 101t
  communication in, 7
    problems of, 99-100
  dynamics of, 101t, 104
  vs. group, 98-99
  as system, 104
Outline, 120
  motivated sequence for, 109-118
  for speeches, 108-109

Pain, 65
Paralanguage, 45t, 48
Patient
  anger demonstration by, 67
  anxiety of, 64, 68
  assessment of, 34, 35
  body motion of, 44

communication with, 4, 20, 53-75
  co-orientation perspective in, 56-58
  social penetration in, 54-56, 55t
as consumer, 58
depressed, 57
interviewing of, 30
  analysis in, 59-61
  configurations for, 63-73
  monitor/observer role in, 64-73
  observer evaluation of, 62
  patient orientation in, 64, 73
  pre-interview evaluation for, 61
  strategies for, 32-33
  implementation of, 32-42
legal rights of, 73
nonverbal communication and, 44
and nurse relationship, 10
  personal distance and, 49
welfare of, 77, 79, 103-104, 120
Peer(s),
  communication with, 79, 80-82
  and interview role, 29
  interviews of, 41t
Perception, 56, 73
Perfume, 49
Personal distance and, 49
Personal greetings, in attention step, 116
Personal space, 48-49, 45t, 48t
Personality, 55
Persuasive interview, 30
Persuasive speech, 107, 108
  motivated sequence for, 109-118
Physician
  communication with, 83-85
  and interview role, 29
  and nurse relationship, 9, 10, 11, 77-78, 96
  personal distance and, 49
Pluckhan, M. L., 4, 24
Pointing step, in need step, 117-118
Pre-interview, evaluation form for, 61
Pre-interview questioning, 29t
Preoutline analysis, 108-109, 111
Preparation, 107
Principles and Types of Speech Communication, 121
Principles of Speech Communication, 122
Probes, 37, 39t
Professionally Speaking: A Concise Guide, 119
Proxemics, 48
Public personal distance, 48, 48t
Public speaking, 7, 106-120, 110, 111, 112-116, 117

  adaptation in, 107
  motivated sequence in, 109-118
    steps in, 116-118
  practicing of, 119
  preparation for, 107
  types of speeches in, 107-108

Questions, 36-39, 39t

Ramification, in need step, 117
Rapport, 58
Reading, of manuscripts, 108
Receiver, of messages, 5, 6
Redding, W. C., 26, 101, 102, 121
Registered nurse, 8
Regulating nonverbal function, 43
Repeating nonverbal function, 43
Report statement, 34, 35
Reprimands, 80-82, 96
Restatements, 37-38, 39t, 67
  as verbal support material, 117
Rhetorical question, 116
Rhetorical Reflector, 17, 18, 22
  implications of, 19
Rhetorical Sensitivity, 17, 18, 19-20, 79, 85
  adaptive behavior and, 31
  implication of, 19
  and interview role, 29
  and professionalism, 21-22, 23
  role-playing and, 63
RHETSEN instrument, 13, 14t-15t, 20t
  implications of, 19-21
  scoring on, 17
Richetto, G., 36, 52
Rickey, J., 26
Rogers, C., 33
Role, clothing and, 49
  of nurse, 4
  within organizations, 101, 101t
  perception of, 7-12
Role-playing, in interviewing exercise, 59-61, 63
Role relationship, clarification of, 85
Rubin, B. D., 121

Satisfaction step, 110, 111, 112, 118
Schedules, for interviews, 40-41
Searight, R., 54
Seating arrangement, 50
Self, 17-18

Sequences, for interviews, 42
Silence, 38, 39t, 67
Smith, D. R., 24
Social-consultative personal distance, 48, 48t, 70
Social penetration process, 54-56, 55t
Specialization, 102
Specific instance, as verbal support material, *117*
Speeches, 107-108
  content of, 118-120
  delivery of, 118-120
  motivated sequence for, 109-118
    steps in, 116-118
  outlining for, 108-109
  practicing of, 119
  presentation of, 120
Statements, 80-81
  in need step, *111, 112*, 116-117
Statistics, as verbal support material, *117*
Status, 49
  hierarchy of, 101t, 102
Stereotype, 35, 46, 70
  of child, 67
Stewart, C. J., 52
Subordinates, 80-82
Substituting nonverbal function, 43
Superiors, 4, 80-82
  interaction with, 20
  and interview role, 29
Supportive behavior, 66, 67, 69, 72
Supportive interview, 30
Sutterley, D. C., 122

Taylor, D., 54
Terminology, 85
  clarification of, 85
Testimony, as verbal support material, *117*
Threats, 82
Touching, 46, 45t
Transaction, 5
Tunnel sequence, 42
Two-party communication, 6, 7

Uniforms, 49

Van de Ven, A., 94, 97
Verbal communication, 5, 6
Verbal support materials, *117*
Visual aids, 120
Visualization step, *110, 112, 116,* 118
Vocal tone, 48
Voice, 119

Watzlawick, P., 6
Williamson, L. K., 24

Yes/no questions, 37, 39t, 41

Zima, J., 36, 52